COPING SUCCESSFULLY WITH ULCERATIVE COLITIS

Peter Cartwright is the former Assistant Director of the National Association for Colitis and Crohn's Disease (NACC). For four years he was responsible for NACC's publications, including the highly regarded member booklet series.

He is the author of *Probiotics for Crohn's and Colitis*, and has spoken at more than 50 local NACC Group meetings on the benefits of probiotics and on the causes of inflammatory bowel disease.

Peter has worked for patient and self-help associations for 17 years, including as National Development Officer with the Self Help Alliance and as Director of the British Stammering Association.

He has an MSc in Microbiology and an MA in Sociology, and is married with two grown-up children.

D0805244

Overcoming Common Problems Series

Selected titles
A full list of titles is available from Sheldon Press,
36 Causton Street, London SW1P 4ST, and on our website at
www.sheldonpress.co.uk

Overcoming Common Problems Series

Overcoming Common Problems Series

Living with Eczema
Jill Eckersley

Living with Fibromyalgia
Christine Craggs-Hinton

Living with Food Intolerance
Alex Gazzola

Living with Grief
Dr Tony Lake

Living with Heart Failure
Susan Elliot-Wright

Living with Loss and Grief
Julia Tugendhat

Living with Lupus
Philippa Pigache

Living with Osteoarthritis
Dr Patricia Gilbert

Living with Osteoporosis
Dr Joan Gomez

Living with Rheumatoid Arthritis
Philippa Pigache

Living with Schizophrenia
Dr Neel Burton and Dr Phil Davison

Living with a Seriously Ill Child
Dr Jan Aldridge

Living with Sjögren's Syndrome
Sue Dyson

Losing a Baby
Sarah Ewing

Losing a Child
Linda Hurcombe

The Multiple Sclerosis Diet Book
Tessa Buckley

Osteoporosis: Prevent and treat
De Tom Smith

Overcoming Agoraphobia
Melissa Murphy

Overcoming Anorexia
Professor J. Hubert Lacey, Christine Craggs-Hinton and Kate Robinson

Overcoming Anxiety
Dr Windy Dryden

Overcoming Back Pain
Dr Tom Smith

Overcoming Depression
Dr Windy Dryden and Sarah Opie

Overcoming Emotional Abuse
Susan Elliot-Wright

Overcoming Hurt
Dr Windy Dryden

Overcoming Insomnia
Susan Elliot-Wright

Overcoming Jealousy
Dr Windy Dryden

Overcoming Procrastination
Dr Windy Dryden

Overcoming Shyness and Social Anxiety
Ruth Searle

Overcoming Tiredness and Exhaustion
Fiona Marshall

The PMS Handbook
Theresa Cheung

Reducing Your Risk of Cancer
Dr Terry Priestman

Safe Dieting for Teens
Linda Ojeda

The Self-Esteem Journal
Alison Waines

Simplify Your Life
Naomi Saunders

Stammering: Advice for all ages
Renée Byrne and Louise Wright

Stress-related Illness
Dr Tim Cantopher

Ten Steps to Positive Living
Dr Windy Dryden

Think Your Way to Happiness
Dr Windy Dryden and Jack Gordon

The Thinking Person's Guide to Happiness
Ruth Searle

Tranquillizers and Antidepressants: When to start them, how to stop
Professor Malcolm Lader

The Traveller's Good Health Guide
Dr Ted Lankester

Treating Arthritis Diet Book
Margaret Hills

Treating Arthritis – The drug-free way
Margaret Hills

Treating Arthritis – More drug-free ways
Margaret Hills

Understanding Obsessions and Compulsions
Dr Frank Tallis

When Someone You Love Has Depression
Barbara Baker

Overcoming Common Problems

Coping Successfully with Ulcerative Colitis

Peter Cartwright

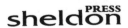

First published in Great Britain in 2004

Sheldon Press
36 Causton Street
London SW1P 4ST

Copyright © Peter Cartwright 2004

British Library Cataloguing-in-Publication Data
A catalogue record for this book is available from the British Library

ISBN 978–0–85969–917–4

3 5 7 9 10 8 6 4

Typeset by Deltatype Limited, Birkenhead, Merseyside
Printed in Great Britain at Ashford Colour Press

Produced on paper from sustainable forests

Contents

Acknowledgements

Many people have helped in the production of this book, in addition to the friendly and talented team at Sheldon Press.

Medical and scientific advice was generously provided by Drs Thomas J. Borody, Isaias Dichi, Stephen Grainger, Mario Guslandi, Stephen Kane, Sunanda Kane and Jeremy Nightingale, and Professors Glenn Gibson and Claudio de Simone. Thanks are also due to Colorectal Nurse Specialist Angie Perrin.

Several people with broad experience of patients' needs also kindly commented on drafts: Maggie Bates, Anne Demick, Stephanie Sadler and Helen Terry.

The quotations from people with ulcerative colitis are given by Nicola Bullock, Liz Byfield, Barbara Coultas, Lynn Driscoll, Elise Dumbleton, Jean Escott, John Fairhurst, Heather Frankcom, Clair Griffiths, Annette Gwinn, Rachel Hayward, Dick Heath, Craig Kershaw, Mrs L. J. Mathers, Myra, Brenda Orlandini, Sarah Parfitt, Sam Pester, Julia Reed, Miss M. Simmonds, Miss Emily Stevens, Mrs A. Maureen Ward, and Mrs Christine Whittle. Their contributions, which improved the book substantially, are much appreciated.

Thanks should go to two friends, who are also freelance editors, for their guidance in making the text much more readable: Loulou Brown and Sara Bernstein.

And finally, many thanks to my wife, Yvonne, for typing substantial parts of the text and for her continual encouragement.

Peter Cartwright

Foreword

I must be one of the few people to have found the diagnosis of ulcerative colitis (UC) rather a relief. My symptoms were, in the late 1960s, initially and wrongly diagnosed as 'gonorrhoea of the rectum', so it's not hard to understand why anything that erased that particularly gruesome idea was a welcome alternative.

I've suffered now for over 30 years and, luckily for me, in a way, my symptoms have slowly got worse and worse, each vile stage creeping up gradually. To find yourself suddenly suffering badly from UC must come as a hideous shock.

Speaking personally, I've never found the feelings of debilitation much of a problem. Lying in bed, with a temperature, unable to eat, and with cramping pains in the stomach – or even having to rush to the loo as you do with gastroenteritis – is unpleasant, but nothing that other people can't identify with. The tiredness, the exhaustion, the faintness, the excruciating pain while on the lavatory – these are all extremely unpleasant, but they are all things that you can, up to a point, share with other people. They can truly say: 'Oh yes, I know how you feel. I remember when I was in Delhi I had the most awful diarrhoea, it was ghastly.'

But there comes a moment when your symptoms start wildly to diverge from those of 'other people'. And that's when it starts to get hairy. First, of course, when people go to the lavatory and look into the pan, they don't usually find a great pool of blood, mucus and gobbets of wobbling bloody jelly. This is an extremely frightening sight. Not everyone has had the really horrible experience of their entire body going into spasms. This means that at the same time you are spurting diarrhoea from one end, you are vomiting from the other. There is no way that I have found of not making my lavatory, at the end of an episode like this, something rather like a dirty protest in the Maze prison. Anyone who has suffered as I have knows how, once poo has got out of control, it gets absolutely every-where – on your hands, on the seat, on the carpet, on your feet . . . even on the walls. (I was once caught short in Schiphol Airport, which was awarded a medal for being the very best airport in the world. Unfortunately, its lavatories were so sophisticated that they would only flush when you walked towards the door, which opened automatically. In order to leave the cubicle spotless – requiring probably about 15 flushings to get clean water – I had to walk to the door 15 times, opening it, and then dart back inside again. The people in the queue were astonished. They must have thought they were starring in *Groundhog Day*.)

Then there are the 'accidents'. I remember one such happening in Brixton market with my son when he was about 10 years old. As I'm a woman who wears tights and – nowadays – always a skirt, an accident can be quite well disguised, although a car is essential. I will never forget driving back home, trying to rise slightly on my seat to stop the stain getting through, with my son, his head out of the window, giggling and holding his nose saying: 'Oh poo! Mum! You stink! Ugh!'

I have learned now, if I go away during an attack, to take a towel to put under me in case of an accident in bed, and a potty just in case I can't get to the bathroom in time. I have learned, too, to snap people's heads off when, on learning what I suffer from, they say: 'Oh, have you tried cutting out wheat?' 'Is it something to do with what you eat?' or 'Have you tried echinacea/ginseng/snake oil?' I simply reply, coldly: 'Doctors have proved that it has absolutely nothing at all to do with diet.'

I have learned, too, to be upfront. 'I have a chronic condition,' I say (the word 'chronic' lets them know that it is with me for ever). 'It is called ulcerative colitis – and it is not to be confused with ordinary colitis since it has, until recently, been life-threatening.' (It's always worth adding this to convey the severity of the condition.) 'It means that I often can't get to the lavatory in time – and when I say get to the lavatory, I am not talking peeing here.' (This is a euphemism, but I'm not of a generation to talk about shit. People get the point.)

I have learned, if I'm out in town, to rush into a shop as soon as I feel the first twinges and ask for a lavatory – and to stay there until the crisis is over, often quite a while. I have learned, as well, that if I'm on a country walk, it is quite okay to say quietly to friends that I'm having a bit of an 'attack' or a 'crisis' and if they would walk on, I'll catch up later. After you've coped with being in the bushes – there's usually a tree or a bush available – you come away feeling rather animal-like and rustic.

I have learned, too, what works for me in the way of medication.

At one point I used to take 20 Salazopyrin® a day, until I stopped once and started again, only nearly to die. My body just couldn't take any more. I have asked my doctor what I can take with what and up to how much, and I have come up with a bizarre and personal combination of medication that seems to work. I have learned, too, that for me UC seems to come on mostly in the spring and always appears after any kind of loss – and to be forewarned is to be forearmed. Once I tell my body that I'm watching it, it doesn't seem to respond quite so predictably.

I have been a lifelong member of the National Association for Colitis and Crohn's Disease, an organization that has kept me up to date with every new medication and provided endless interest in its letters pages. Sharing experiences with other people through the newsletter has been extremely helpful for me, particularly knowing, too, that while for some people UC can be totally disabling, for others it can be overcome. I have always refused to let it get the better of me, except twice when it sent me into hospital for a month each time. If I stayed indoors simply because I might have an accident, then, I feel, my life would be over. In my rush for the loo I once even defied the orders of an air steward who assured me that if I left my seat as the plane was landing, it would have be diverted to another airport, holding up flights all over the world. I told him not to be so stupid and went anyway. We landed.

I only wish this marvellous book had been out when I was younger. It is an invaluable resource for people with UC – always Crohn's poor younger sister I have felt, the Cinderella of the world of inflammatory bowel disease. It is packed with useful facts, tips, information and explanations. Armed with this book, a bit of courage and a determination never to let life be dominated by embarrassment, those with UC have nothing to fear.

Virginia Ironside

Introduction: basics of ulcerative colitis

This book is written for people with ulcerative colitis (UC), their family members and close friends. It aims to give clear and readable information about UC, to explain how to reduce the effects of UC on daily life, and to describe the potential of new treatments. Together with Crohn's disease, a similar ailment, UC is referred to as an inflammatory bowel disease, but this book focuses on UC alone.

What is ulcerative colitis?

Ulcerative colitis is an illness in which part of the intestine becomes inflamed and develops ulcers (open sores). The part of the intestine affected by UC is the colon (also known as the large intestine), which forms the lower end of the digestive tube. It is the inner lining of the colon that is inflamed in UC.

The colon removes water from undigested food so that the waste matter becomes more solid. In people with UC the inflamed lining of the colon is less efficient at absorbing water so that the contents of the lower intestine remain liquid. Diarrhoea develops from the liquid waste and this may be very difficult to control.

In addition to severe and persistent diarrhoea, people with UC may also find blood, mucus and pus in their stools (faeces).

- The blood is present because the ulcers on the intestine damage the lining, which leads to bleeding.
- Mucus is a slimy substance that lines the intestine. It protects the intestine from hard food and harmful germs and helps to lubricate the movement of the contents of the intestine. When the intestine is inflamed, as in UC, mucus is shed and the tissues of the intestine produce a lot more as a replacement. As the inflammation in UC tends to be continual, newly produced mucus often comes out with the diarrhoea and blood.
- Pus, which is a thick yellow or green liquid, may also be produced in UC. The pus consists of white blood cells that are

part of the inflammatory process, plus dead bacteria if there is any infection in the ulcers.

Other symptoms of UC may include crampy abdominal pain, tiredness and fever. Less commonly there may be skin complaints or inflammation of the eyes, the mouth or the joints.

About half of all people with UC have only the lowest end of the colon affected. The symptoms are usually mild diarrhoea with blood and mucus in the stool and frequent false urges (tenesmus) to have a bowel motion. Occasionally, bleeding with constipation occurs instead of diarrhoea. In other people, the inflammation extends up the colon from the rectum, sometimes affecting the whole colon. Usually, the more extensive the disease, the more severe and diverse the symptoms.

One of the main practical concerns for people with UC is having an episode of bowel incontinence. The urge to empty the bowels may be sudden and very strong. There may be difficulty in quickly finding a toilet, and at night, sleep may be disturbed by strong diarrhoea urges. Personal and social confidence may be affected by the fear of having an 'accident'.

Liz

I was losing weight, and the bleeding and diarrhoea were getting worse, up to 10 times a day and uncontrollable. There were many times when I had 'accidents' while I was out in shops or driving and also while I was at home. Although I live on my own and no one else knew about these 'accidents', I found them very traumatic.

In the UK, there are about 90,000 people with UC. It most commonly starts during young adulthood, although it may start at any age.

UC is not infectious. You cannot catch it from someone else or give it to someone else.

Use of the word 'colitis'

Colitis is a general term that means inflammation of the colon. It is also used in common parlance to cover such conditions as irritable bowel syndrome (IBS) or gastroenteritis (infectious diarrhoea). Ulcerative colitis is a completely separate disease that is usually more serious and troublesome than these other forms of 'colitis'.

What causes ulcerative colitis?

The cause of UC is currently not known, but the prevalence of the disease in different populations indicates that it is caused by a combination of environmental and genetic factors. The main theories about the disease are described in Chapter 1. There are also descriptions of the digestive system, the colon and the role of the gut microflora (resident bacteria in the intestine).

How is UC diagnosed and monitored?

It can be difficult, initially, to diagnose UC. There is a wide range of explanations for persistent diarrhoea and most of these illnesses are more common than UC.

A number of different tests may be undertaken to help reach a diagnosis. The most useful is an endoscopy, whereby a tube is placed into the back passage to enable the doctor to examine the rectum and colon. Other tests include X-ray pictures and various blood tests.

After diagnosis, some of these tests will be repeated periodically to check how the disease is progressing. The tests and examinations will enable your doctor to inform you how much of the colon is affected by inflammation. Chapter 2 explains more fully the process of diagnosis and the tests involved.

What are the treatments available?

Currently there is no cure for UC. Instead, it is treated with a range of drugs, and these may be effective in bringing the disease under control. The effectiveness of drugs varies from person to person, depending mainly on the severity of the condition. UC is a fluctuating illness, in that there are periods when it is active (flare-ups), and other times when it is quiescent (in remission). It is not possible to predict how fluctuations will proceed. Information on different drug treatments is given in Chapter 3.

Is there a recommended diet?

People who are recently diagnosed usually ask their doctor or nurse whether there is a particular diet that should be followed. Unfortunately, there is no recommended diet, because medical research has not shown that a particular diet works to reduce disease.

The food you eat is not irrelevant, however. Good nutrition is important to help the body cope with the effect of continuing inflammation. The amount of fibre in the diet is also important. A small proportion of people with UC are intolerant of certain foods and feel better if they avoid them. These matters are covered in Chapter 4.

What are the day-to-day problems with UC?

The difficulties associated with daily living are connected to:

- adjustments to the continuing nature of the condition;
- worries about the long-term effects of UC, including side effects of the medications, complications such as colon cancer, a continuing lack of energy and fears about possible surgery;
- effects on personal relationships as the result of an embarrassing condition, which may be hard to discuss; and
- coping with practical issues relating to persistent diarrhoea.

All these concerns are discussed in detail in Chapter 5.

Non-intestinal complications

A small proportion of people with UC also have health problems that are associated with it. These may include inflammation of the joints and skin conditions. The full range of possible complications is described in Chapter 6.

Is surgery sometimes needed?

If the UC is severe and has intolerable effects on a person's life, the doctor may propose that the whole of the colon be surgically removed. This is known as a colectomy. UC only affects the colon, including the rectum, so it cannot return if the colon is removed. Another reason for a colectomy is the discovery of signs of cancer in the colon or rectum (or pre-cancerous signs). Also, if the UC causes very rapid deterioration of the gut, a rare occurrence, an emergency colectomy will be needed. Chapter 7 discusses these matters, the types of surgery available, and the practical details of being hospitalized both before and after the operation.

If your colon has to be removed, there is usually a choice between having an ileostomy or an internal pouch to deal with bodily waste. Chapter 8 describes these alternatives.

Only a minority of people with UC require surgery, but those that do usually report that they feel much better afterwards.

Special circumstances

The treatment of children with UC is somewhat different to that of adults. A major concern is for the child's growth. The inflammation itself, plus the effect of some medications, together with a reluctance on the part of the child to eat may lead to a delay in physical development. The medical team may recommend a special dietary approach.

Another area of special consideration is fertility and pregnancy. For women with UC, it is perfectly possible to have a successful pregnancy. There are usually worries about the effect of medications on the baby, but it is generally considered safer to keep the UC under control with the continued use of medication than to stop taking the drugs.

These two matters are discussed in Chapter 9, along with issues that specifically concern the over-60s.

Probiotics and prebiotics

One of the most promising areas of future treatment lies with probiotics and prebiotics. The former are products containing beneficial bacteria, and the latter are types of soluble dietary fibre that stimulate an increase in numbers of beneficial bacteria in the intestine.

It is known that the gut microflora play an important role in the continued inflammation of UC, and that people with UC have a smaller proportion of beneficial bacteria on the lining of the colon than the general population. There is growing evidence that by taking probiotics a better balance of bacteria in the microflora may be achieved, together with a reduction in the severity of UC. Prebiotics may be able to increase the numbers of beneficial bacteria already living in the intestine. Chapter 10 gives up-to-date information on this new area of research.

What does the future offer?

Molecular biology is an important scientific advance that uses special techniques to analyse the molecules and chemical processes in cells. The increased knowledge gained from the use of these techniques is likely to lead to identification of the genes involved in UC, as well as an acceleration in the development of a new wave of drugs.

Another area that may lead to greater knowledge is examination of the effect of nicotine on UC. People with UC who smoke tend to have a less severe version of the disease. It is believed that the active ingredient in tobacco in this regard is probably nicotine, and investigations into this field may explain why this is happening. There may also be more research into the benefits of nicotine patches.

There is some evidence that certain ingredients of fish oil have anti-inflammatory effects on active UC if the oil is consumed in large quantities. Further research may show whether fish oil has the potential for being a new treatment for UC inflammation.

About one-third of people with UC believe that stress can cause a flare-up of their disease. There is potential for examining what is happening to such people. Also, guidance on coping with excessive stress may be helpful.

All these matters are covered in Chapter 11, together with two unusual experimental developments, parasitic worms and faecal enemas, which indicate how solutions to the problem of UC are being approached from many directions.

Throughout this book, I have inserted anecdotes from people who have UC. These quotes provide details of their personal experiences with diagnosis, treatment and daily life. They are meant to give you some indication of the variety of experiences of people who live with UC. Perhaps you will relate to some of them more than others. Remember what works for one person may not work for you. Each person's story, including your own, is unique.

1

What causes ulcerative colitis?

Doctors first identified UC in the late nineteenth century. The number of diagnosed cases of the disease increased substantially in the twentieth century. Statistics suggest that the increase in the annual numbers of new UC cases levelled out from around 1970, although the incidence of proctitis (UC affecting the rectum only) may have continued to rise. Now in the twenty-first century in the UK, one person in about 650 has UC, and each year about 6000 new cases are diagnosed.

Maureen
I was diagnosed in 1960 when I was 16. At that time UC was almost unheard of. Because I was suffering dreadful pains in my joints, it was originally misdiagnosed as rheumatic fever.

The cause of UC remains unknown, but characteristics of the disease in different populations may indicate likely risk factors.

UC is associated with industrialized, urban and developed areas, especially in North America, Scandinavia and western Europe. There are very few cases of UC in poor and underdeveloped countries. African–Americans have a higher incidence of UC than Africans living in Africa. Similarly, there is higher incidence of the disease among British Asians than among Asians living in India, and Jews in the United States have a higher rate of cases than Israeli Jews. This pattern suggests an 'environmental trigger', which is a term that covers a large range of possibilities (for example, a pollutant in the air, food or water; changes in diet; differences of lifestyle). However, this explanation is not much help in identifying the cause unless the specific environmental factor can be identified.

There are indicators that a genetic element is also involved in the cause. In some families, UC (and Crohn's disease) seem to occur fairly frequently. Furthermore, studies of identical twins (those that have exactly the same genes as each other) have shown that when one twin develops UC, the other has about a 15-per-cent chance of also developing the disease. In Western countries, the proportion in the general population who develop UC is approximately 0.2 per

1

cent. Thus the studies of identical twins confirm that there is a genetic element in the development of UC.

UC therefore appears to be caused by environmental factors, as yet unknown, in individuals who have a genetic susceptibility.

The main environmental theories

There are three main theories as to why UC is more common in the UK, Europe and North America.

The first is the 'hygiene theory', whereby it is suggested that children develop a poor immune system (the body's defence system) because they are raised in a hygienic environment. Improved hygiene over the past century has helped to reduce infant mortality dramatically, but this may prove to be a drawback for some children. With fewer viruses, bacteria and parasites reaching the intestine and stimulating gut immune cells, the immune system may not develop as well as in previous generations. This may make people more susceptible to developing UC.

There is also a 'dietary theory'. This theory suggests that the food produced and consumed in Western countries increases the likelihood of developing UC. It might be that particular foods encourage different types of gut bacteria and that these have a different effect on the immune cells in the colon.

A third theory relates to harmful microbes. This suggests that a specific bacterium or virus (that may be more prevalent in Western environments) is the cause of UC and continues to stimulate the inflammation.

None of these three theories has been proven. It is possible that all three have played a part in the increased incidence of UC.

Knowing about UC

Although the cause of UC is currently unknown, nevertheless a great deal has been discovered about the disease over the past 40 years. If you have a chronic (long-term) condition, such as UC, you can benefit substantially from knowing about your disease. Not only will your greater knowledge allow you to discuss fully your circumstances with your doctor, but it will also help you to cope with the challenges of day-to-day life.

The digestive system

As UC is a disease of the digestive system, it is essential to have an understanding of the main elements involved in digesting food. We eat food for the growth and repair of the body and to gain energy. For this to take place food needs to be broken down and absorbed into the body, a process known as digestion. Digestion takes place in a tube that runs from the mouth to the anus. The whole of the digestive tube is known as the alimentary canal, and from the stomach onwards it is known as the intestine.

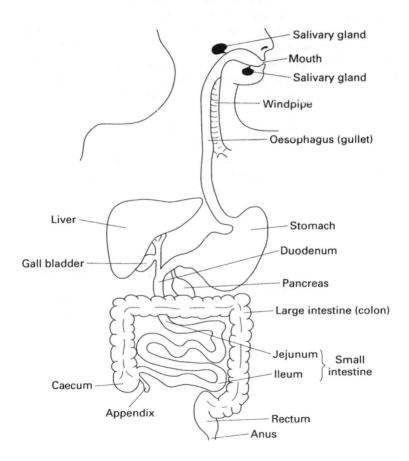

Figure 1: The digestive system

The digestive process

The digestive process starts in the mouth where food is chewed to break it down into smaller pieces. Liquid (saliva) from the mouth is mixed with the food. The saliva contains enzymes – chemicals that assist the breakdown of complex molecules of food into simpler molecules.

From the mouth, the food passes down a straight tube (the oesophagus) into the stomach. The stomach is a bag-shaped organ in which the food is stored for one to two hours while it is churned by the movement of the stomach muscles. Acid and other enzymes are secreted from the stomach wall to break down the food even further.

By the time the food leaves the stomach to enter the small intestine, it has become liquefied and is called chyme. The first part of the small intestine is the duodenum. Various digestive juices from the liver and pancreas are added to the chyme in the duodenum. These juices neutralize the acid from the stomach so that the small intestine is not damaged.

The chyme passes along the small intestine, which in most people has a length of between six and seven metres. (It is from the small bore of the tube, not from its length, that the small intestine gets its name.) In the small intestine digestion is completed and tiny molecules in the chyme are absorbed into the body by passing

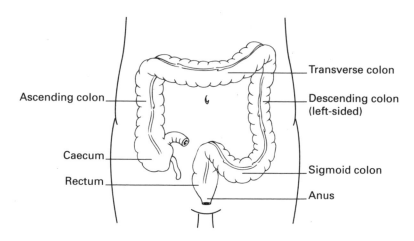

Figure 2: The colon (large intestine)

through the intestine wall and into the blood vessels. Once in the bloodstream the nutritious molecules can travel anywhere they are needed in the body.

The colon starts at the end of the small intestine, and this is the part of the intestine affected by UC. The beginning of the colon is known as the caecum. This leads to the ascending colon, then the transverse colon, the descending colon, the sigmoid colon, and finally to the rectum.

The function of the colon

For a long time it was thought that the colon was a relatively unimportant part of the body. The colon absorbs water from the faeces (undigested chyme) so that the body has plenty of fluid. As it does so, the faeces turn into more solid stools, which can be passed out through the anus in a controlled way. Some salts are also absorbed with the water; the salts are useful for the normal functioning of human cells and tissues.

For a relatively simple organ, the colon is prone to quite a lot of disease. For example, colon cancer is one of the most common forms of cancer. Furthermore, irritable bowel syndrome and diverticulitis are two very common illnesses that involve the colon. Also, many people find that they suffer regularly from constipation or diarrhoea that originate in the colon.

More recently, attention has been given to the role of bacteria in the colon. There are hundreds of billions of bacteria that reside in the colon, known collectively as microflora. There are more bacterial cells in the colon than there are human cells in the body. Everyone has his or her own unique mix of bacteria in the microflora which develops from infancy. Much is still unknown about these resident bacteria, but it is now recognized that they play some positive roles. The most important is known as 'colonization resistance', whereby the microflora make it difficult for harmful microbes to become established in the intestine and cause infection in the body. The microflora also produce a wide range of chemicals, some of which help to improve the health of the colon lining.

Some of the resident bacteria may, however, have negative consequences, and one of these is to stimulate the continuation of inflammation caused by UC.

How the gut microflora stimulate UC inflammation

Inflammation is an important part of the processes involved in defending the body from infection by harmful microbes (viruses, bacteria, parasites and fungi). All of the different processes that the body undertakes to defend itself from microbes, together with the related cells and tissues, are known collectively as the immune system.

The immune system is a complex system, but the basics can be understood quite easily. A large proportion of the immune cells are found in the intestine. This is not surprising, because while the intestine has to absorb nutrients, it also has to keep out harmful microbes. It is important to distinguish quickly the good from the bad. The immune cells are present in the intestinal wall ready to attack harmful microbes and ignore beneficial food particles.

It is extraordinary that the gut immune system can also distinguish harmless resident bacteria in the intestine from harmful newly arrived bacteria. It is not known how this is achieved. What is known, however, is that people with UC have an immune system that has become confused between the good and the bad bacteria. Their gut immune system reacts to harmless resident bacteria of the colon as if they were harmful invaders. The immune system sends certain white blood cells to the point of invasion to destroy the invaders. In order to get the white blood cells quickly to the point of battle inflammation takes place.

Inflammation is a process in which the area is flooded with blood. The gaps between tissue cells alter so that blood can flow easily towards the point of invasion but cannot easily flow away. An example of inflammation can be seen when you have a small cut on the surface of a finger. If the cut is not cleaned and covered, the skin in the area will become red, swollen and tender. This is because microbes have entered the broken skin and triggered an inflammatory response. Blood has flowed to the area so that white blood cells can destroy the microbes.

In the colon, once UC has started, the resident gut bacteria become mistakenly identified by the immune system as the enemy, and the inflammation continues. In most battles, in addition to the combatants dying or being wounded, the local area is damaged. The same is true with the process of inflammation. Damage occurs to the tissues of the colon, in the form of ulceration, and this leads to the symptoms of UC.

6

The inflammation continues because the gut microflora are always present and are continually stimulating the immune system into attack mode.

What is not clear in explaining UC is:

- how it initially starts;
- why it fluctuates from flare-ups to remission and back again;
- whether the main problem lies with the types of bacteria resident in the intestine, the poor functioning of the immune system or a fault in the mechanism for repairing the damaged lining of the colon;
- what role genes play in making the immune system react incorrectly.

Scientific research into UC is continuing, and it is only a matter of time (and money) before the cause is uncovered. Further information on future developments can be found in Chapters 10 and 11.

2

Diagnosis and tests

The symptoms of UC may appear suddenly or gradually. The methods used for diagnosis are essentially the same whatever the symptoms, but they vary somewhat depending on the severity of the disease.

If symptoms appear gradually, it may take quite a long time to confirm the diagnosis. The reasons for this are twofold. First, it is not possible for the doctor to discover solely by an external physical examination what is causing the trouble inside the body. Secondly, diarrhoea is a symptom for a number of different illnesses, many of which are more common than UC. The doctor will look for more usual diseases first and only then, if the diagnosis proves negative for these, will he or she move on to consider the less common conditions. Occasionally, there is a long delay in confirming diagnosis.

Elise

I began to experience symptoms of bloating, pain and diarrhoea. I had just turned 17 and was doing my first year of A-levels at school and because my GP believed that I was suffering from exam-related stress, he immediately diagnosed me with irritable bowel syndrome (IBS).

After about a year of living with symptoms that were spiralling out of control, I managed to persuade my GP to refer me to a gastroenterologist. However, after a quick look with a sigmoidoscope he informed me that there was absolutely nothing wrong with me and suggested that I enrol on a 'stress busters' course.

I started university, and by then was going to the toilet up to 20 times a day (and at night), was extremely tired all the time and had started to pass blood. I also suffered lots of panic attacks. A year later I succeeded again in persuading my GP to let me see another gastroenterologist. This time I went privately, because on the NHS there would be a long wait, because according to my GP my case was not urgent! This time I thought that I really would get somewhere, but another sigmoidoscope later, I received another IBS diagnosis.

By now I was sometimes incontinent and I referred myself to a specialist; this time an allergy specialist (I was getting desperate). A year later, the appointment came through. At last, someone took me seriously: he rushed through an appointment for me with another gastroenterologist and she referred me for all the necessary tests the following week. I was finally started on medication for a disease that I had never heard of called ulcerative colitis.

Elise's story is unusual, as the great majority of people with UC will have their disease identified by sigmoidoscopy (see endoscopy, page 12) at a hospital outpatient clinic.

Case history

When you report an illness to your doctor, the first thing he or she will do is ask questions about the symptoms. The doctor will want you to describe what is wrong, in your own words. This can create a problem – how to talk about UC without feeling embarrassed.

Saying you have an 'upset tummy' or 'stomach trouble' will not be enough. The doctor will want to know more precisely what you mean by this. It is therefore worth planning how you will describe the symptoms. How will you describe bodily waste? While urine is a commonly used word and 'pee' is slang, both words are reasonably acceptable in public. What should you use to describe the solid waste? The words 'poo', 'shit', 'faeces' or 'stools' are all options for getting your point across to the doctor. In this book, I will mainly use the word 'stools'. What about describing the process of passing the solid waste? While doctors may use 'defaecation' when talking among themselves, 'passing stools' or 'having a bowel motion' might be more comfortable alternatives for you.

There is also the difficulty of describing the part of the body involved. The word 'bottom', like the word 'tummy', is a bit vague. There may be no alternative but to use the technical terms of 'anus' and 'rectum'. However, 'back passage' is frequently used to describe both anus and rectum together.

Whatever words you use, please remember that doctors are very unlikely to be embarrassed. They have heard it all before! The most important point to remember is to describe your symptoms as accurately as possible. Don't leave something out just because describing it may make you embarrassed. Your health is far more important than a bit of social discomfort.

If speaking about bowels is really too embarrassing, you could take a friend or partner with you to explain. Or you could write everything down in a note to give to your doctor.

The symptoms that your doctor may be most interested in are the frequency with which you pass stools (or diarrhoea), including during the night. The doctor will also want to know what your stools look like, and if there is any blood passed. He or she may seek further information, such as whether you feel that something specific started the symptoms, whether these symptoms have occurred before and whether any of your relatives have suffered similar symptoms.

Initial physical examination

Your doctor may also examine your body. In the case of persistent diarrhoea and pain, this may involve using the hands to feel the abdomen (tummy area) for tenderness and any unusual lumps. The doctor also may feel for any unusual lumps or shapes, such as haemorrhoids (piles), by putting a finger into your rectum. The doctor will wear a thin latex glove with lubricant placed on the finger. Although this may sound somewhat alarming and invasive, this particular investigative technique should not cause great discomfort. Also, please remember that all investigations by doctors can only take place with your consent.

You may be asked to return, with a stool sample in a container supplied by the doctor. The appearance of the sample will be examined, and some of it will be sent to a laboratory for testing.

Common causes of diarrhoea

Basically, diarrhoea occurs either as a result of the body trying to flush out harmful germs or substances or because not enough water is being absorbed from the intestine into the body to allow firm stools to form.

The most common explanation for severe diarrhoea is an infection caused by a bacterium or virus. Testing a stool sample is aimed at discovering if there is an infectious microbe present. Infectious diarrhoea, also known as gastroenteritis, is usually caused by bacteria, such as *Campylobacter, Shigella* or *Salmonella*. Symptoms arising from these infections normally cease within three or four days. Some cases, however, can be persistent, so it cannot be assumed that just because the diarrhoea has lasted a long time it is not a form of gastroenteritis.

Another common explanation for diarrhoea is irritable bowel syndrome (IBS). In IBS the surface of the colon appears perfectly normal. The colon muscles go into spasm and this interrupts the normal function of the intestine, often causing diarrhoea alternating with constipation.

Other possible diagnoses for diarrhoea and blood in the stool include certain sexually transmitted diseases and cancer of the colon. Fear of colon cancer often drives people to visit their doctor when they find blood in their stool, although they may have had persistent diarrhoea for some time.

Investigations and tests

If analysis of the stool sample does not show an infectious bacterium or virus as the cause of diarrhoea, further tests are needed. Doctors use a variety of methods to reach a diagnosis. The main ones are:

- endoscopy (the passing of a tube up the back passage);
- taking X-ray pictures; and
- taking blood samples.

Lynn
The thought of investigations was daunting ... A lady doctor examined me; she was very understanding and thorough. She gave me lots of relevant information ... Off I went for X-ray, and blood tests, not to mention the personal examinations. I know they have to be done, but I realize how important privacy and dignity are, now that I have been put into that situation.

Investigations are not pleasant, as we don't talk about that part of the anatomy. You feel like the whole hospital has seen parts of your body that you yourself will never see. You have to be forward thinking and not let it get you down, otherwise you feel worse than before.

Endoscopy

An endoscope is a slim, tube-shaped piece of equipment with a light at one end to enable the doctor to look inside the body. For suspected UC, the endoscope used is either a sigmoidoscope or a colonoscope.

A sigmoidoscope is either a rigid or flexible tube and is long enough to pass into the rectum, enabling the doctor to see as far as the sigmoid colon (the lowest part of the colon). As the rectum is almost always affected in UC, it is a good way of diagnosing the disease. The sigmoidoscopy procedure takes between five and 20 minutes, and there is usually only mild discomfort.

A colonoscope is an endoscope that is long enough to travel the whole length of the colon and has a camera at one end. It is used to confirm the diagnosis and to assess how much of the colon is inflamed. It also shows how severe the inflammation is. The procedure usually takes between 15 and 30 minutes. Other abnormalities can also be observed, such as narrowings or widenings of the colon, or early signs of cancerous growths. A colonoscopy will not be undertaken if disease symptoms are severe. The disease will need to be brought under control first.

A healthy colon has a mucosa (lining) that is smooth and pink in appearance, but in UC the lining has a granular (bumpy) appearance, is reddened and raw-looking and bruises easily. There may also be oedema (excess watery fluid) in the lining. In more severe cases of the disease, bleeding of the mucosa will be seen, together with pus and excessive mucus. Unlike Crohn's disease, where inflammation may appear in patches, inflammation in UC is continuous. It is almost always present in the rectum and often in at least part of the colon. The length of colon affected varies with the individual.

A colonoscope allows pictures to be taken so that they can be examined later on. In addition to a light and camera at the end of the tube, there is also a little gadget that can take a very small piece (biopsy) from the intestinal wall that can be examined in the laboratory. The appearance of the cells under the microscope can show whether they are affected by UC or by another inflammatory bowel disease (such as Crohn's disease), or whether they are cancerous or normal.

For the colonoscope to give a clear picture, it is necessary to clean out the contents of the colon. There will always be some faecal residue that makes it difficult to examine the colon clearly, even if the person concerned has diarrhoea. The patient must stop eating for up to two days beforehand and only drink clear fluids. A special bowel cleansing solution (such as Picolax® or Klean-Prep®) is drunk, which provokes severe diarrhoea. Most people find this painless, although a few suffer crampy pains.

The colonoscopy process itself can be uncomfortable but is rarely painful. If you undergo this procedure, you will usually be mildly sedated to reduce anxiety and discomfort. You will therefore not be able to drive safely immediately afterwards, or operate machinery or consume alcohol. There is also a very small risk of the intestine wall being perforated. This risk is kept to an absolute minimum by careful training for the health professional who undertakes this procedure (usually a doctor).

Endoscopies are the best tool for diagnosis. Even so, it is not always possible to confirm that UC is present. In approximately 10 per cent of cases of inflamed colon a diagnosis of 'indeterminate colitis' is given, because it is not possible to distinguish UC from Crohn's disease.

X-rays

While the use of an endoscope is the best tool for diagnosis, its use is not always effective or appropriate. For example, if the disease is very severe, the bowel cleansing would cause too much discomfort, and the insertion of the tube into the rectum would be too unpleasant. Even if the diarrhoea is relatively mild or in remission, the colon may have become narrowed so that the endoscope tube cannot pass as far as required. Under these circumstances, X-ray pictures may help with the diagnosis.

Simple X-ray pictures of the chest and abdomen will provide some information. The intestine is soft tissue and is not normally shown using X-rays. However, if there is gas or some faecal residue this will show up. It should be possible to see if the colon has become dilated or if there is something else substantially abnormal, such as oedema or deep ulceration.

Barium is a chemical that can be used to make the soft-tissue visible on X-ray film. A liquid version of the barium (a barium meal) is swallowed and, as it lines the intestine, X-ray pictures are taken over several hours. Bowel preparation is not needed, but the patient has to stop eating or drinking for 10 hours beforehand.

An alternative to swallowing barium is to have it passed into the back passage. After bowel cleansing, as for colonoscopy, a tube is inserted into the rectum and liquid barium is poured into the colon. Air is usually added so that the colon is widened and a better picture obtained. The patient moves into different positions to help ensure that the barium liquid coats the whole of the colon, and X-ray pictures are taken while different positions are held. This procedure takes about 20 minutes in total.

The drawbacks with the use of barium are that:

- barium meal is a thick liquid and can be unpleasant to swallow;
- a barium enema may give a strong urge to empty the bowel, and this urge has to be resisted;
- the addition of air to the barium enema, which gives much better clarity of detail, may cause cramping abdominal pain and carries with it an increased risk of perforation or dilatation of the colon; and
- for a couple of days afterwards the stools turn pale and may be difficult to flush away in the toilet, because they are coated with barium. There may also be a tendency to develop constipation, so a gentle laxative may be prescribed by your doctor.

Blood tests

A third type of investigation involves taking samples of blood. A sample is taken from a vein in the arm, and various laboratory tests are performed on the blood. The tests look for the numbers of white blood cells and other cells associated with inflammation, the number of red blood cells, and the amount of haemoglobin (to look for anaemia).

Other tests check for shortages of vitamins and minerals, including iron. Yet another test checks for various enzymes that indicate the health of the liver, and for shortages of proteins such as albumin. All these various blood tests provide useful information about the likely explanation for the diarrhoea.

Occasionally, a radio-labelled leucocyte scan is undertaken. Here, a sample of your blood has a very small amount of radioactive substance added to the leucocytes (white blood cells). The blood is re-injected into the blood stream and the white cells are attracted to the areas of inflammation. A special type of camera that is sensitive to radioactivity can then provide a picture of the parts of the intestine that are inflamed.

Nicola
The diarrhoea started up again, I was bleeding from my anus when going to the toilet, was off my food and had crippling stomach pains . . . Again I went back and saw a different doctor, who examined me, and said she was going to make a hospital appointment for me to be looked at properly. That same afternoon the hospital rang and said they could see me straight away. When I got there a consultant came to see me and wanted to do a sigmoidoscopy there and then. After doing so, they decided to keep me in hospital. I had to use a stool chart to record every time I went to the toilet and how much I was passing to see if it was improving. A few days later I was sent to have a colonoscopy done. I was knocked out at the time so didn't feel a thing. I was just a bit windy afterwards.

Some days later, I had some X-rays done to see if the inflammation of my bowel had changed. I was also sent to have a white blood cell test, which they did to check if it was definitely ulcerative colitis that I had, and not anything else. A nurse removed some blood from me and the white cells were tagged and then put back into my bloodstream. The white cells then moved around the body and because they were tagged they showed up which bits were inflamed. The test confirmed that I had got ulcerative colitis.

After diagnosis

Blood tests are useful in monitoring progress of the disease, and therefore may be undertaken regularly, depending on your circumstances. For example, in those receiving immunosuppressant drugs, such as azathioprine (Imuran®), it is important to check that the numbers of blood cells are not falling.

Endoscopies are also to be expected during the treatment and monitoring of UC, as they provide the best method for examining the inflammation. The frequency with which you have an endoscopy (either a sigmoidoscopy or a colonoscopy) will depend on the nature of your UC and on the policy of your hospital.

15

Barium X-rays may also take place occasionally as part of the monitoring process, but usually much less frequently than endoscopies and blood tests.

Types of UC

When a diagnosis of UC has been confirmed, it is likely that your doctor will be able to describe the type of UC you have. Different portions of the colon can be diseased, from the rectum extending up the colon. In some people the portion affected is static, while in others it progresses along the colon over time. For example, up to 30 per cent of people whose UC is limited to the rectum will find that, with time, the inflammation will extend further along the colon.

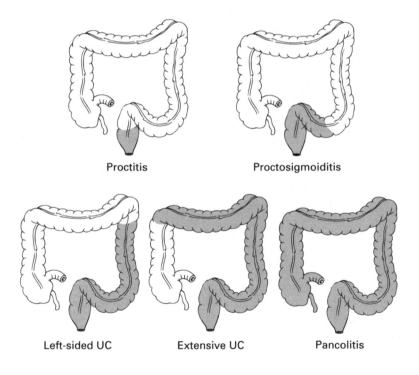

Proctitis   Proctosigmoiditis

Left-sided UC   Extensive UC   Pancolitis

Figure 3: Different areas of the colon affected

Proctitis is the name given to UC in which only the rectum is affected. Proctosigmoiditis is inflammation of the rectum and the sigmoid colon. Left-sided UC involves inflammation from the rectum all the way up the left side of the colon. Extensive UC usually refers to the colon being affected along the transverse colon, and pancolitis is inflammation of the entire colon. In general terms, the disease is more severe the more of the colon affected. Sometimes, however, severe symptoms are experienced by people with proctosigmoiditis, while in a small number of people with pancolitis few symptoms are experienced.

3

Treatments

Treatments currently available for UC aim to stop the diarrhoea, reduce the level of inflammation and keep the symptoms in remission. At present, the disease cannot be cured because the cause of UC is not properly understood. Some surgeons describe a total colectomy (the complete removal of the colon) as a 'cure', but since this is major surgery involving considerable lifestyle adjustments, it is not what most people mean when they say they are looking for a cure.

Once the diagnosis of UC has been given, it is initially quite common to feel great relief that it is not colon cancer. Subsequently, however, it can be quite depressing to think about having a disease that is not currently curable and for which you may have to take medication for the rest of your life.

Knowing about the treatments will, however, assist you in maximizing the opportunities to lessen the disease and its effects on your daily life. The main treatment route is through the use of pharmaceutical drugs. When the disease first appears, and whenever it flares up again, the main type of drug used to bring it under control is the corticosteroid.

Corticosteroids

Corticosteroids are a type of hormone (a chemical that stimulates body cells and tissues) produced by the adrenal glands, which are situated just above the kidneys. Although corticosteroids are often referred to simply as 'steroids', they are not the same as anabolic steroids, which strengthen muscles and have become notorious through their misuse by certain athletes.

The main corticosteroid, naturally produced by the human body, is hydrocortisone (also known as cortisol). It affects blood pressure and salt and sugar levels, and is produced in greater quantities at times of stress.

In the past, severe cases of ulcerative colitis used to carry a risk of death. There was no reliable treatment to bring the inflammation under control, and the body was unable to recover from the cumulative effects of severe disease. With the introduction of corticosteroids, however, the number of people dying from UC plummeted. Nowadays the risk of death for people with UC is only marginally higher than for the general population.

In the middle of the twentieth century, it was discovered that hydrocortisone, if provided in larger quantities than that naturally produced by the body, had the effect of reducing the redness, swelling and pain of inflammation. Doctors started to use this particular hormone as a treatment for rheumatism. Subsequently, it was used to treat UC and proved to be a major breakthrough in treatment. It is not known exactly how corticosteroids bring inflammation under control, but through clinical trials and through their use by doctors for more than 40 years, they have been shown to work very effectively.

While hydrocortisone is still used in the treatment of UC, it is now more common to use a manufactured corticosteroid called prednisolone (or, in the USA, a very similar compound called prednisone).

Corticosteroids are the main drug used to bring an acute attack (flare-up) under control. Initially a high dose is given and gradually the dose is reduced as the symptoms subside. The aim is to reduce steroid dosage until it is stopped altogether. This is because:

- steroids may cause a number of unpleasant side effects, including the weakening of bones;
- long-term use of steroids makes the body reduce its natural production of hydrocortisone; and
- steroids cause reduced immunity from infection.

Margaret
I was diagnosed with UC at the age of 51, following a colonoscopy. I was put on intravenous steroids and kept in hospital for 6 weeks. On returning home, I was given a different drug. It has been 15 months since I was in hospital and currently I am feeling well. I am due to have a bone scan in July and have been informed that I have brittle bones in my spine due to steroid use.

Despite these difficulties, for most people with UC, steroids are the best drugs to get the disease under control quickly.

If you have a very severe attack of diarrhoea and bleeding caused by the disease and you have to be taken into hospital, then it is very likely that you will be given steroids intravenously (injected directly into a vein). This is usually more effective than oral steroids, probably because a higher dose reaches the tissues of the colon.

If your UC symptoms are less severe, steroids may be administered as a tablet or as a rectal enema. Steroid enemas are recommended for people whose UC affects no more than the rectum and the sigmoid colon. This is known as 'topical' administration (meaning that the medication is applied directly to a part of the body). The alternative is a 'systemic' drug that is taken by mouth and enters the bloodstream via the small intestine and passes around the body affecting many parts, including the inflamed colon. Adding a steroid via the back passage leads to fewer side effects. This is because more of the steroid reaches the target area (the lining of the colon) with less entering the bloodstream to affect other parts of the body. It also means that lower doses of steroids may be used than with steroids taken by mouth while still having the same effect.

For some people, the idea of inserting a tube into the rectum, on a daily basis, is too awkward, unpleasant and embarrassing to contemplate. But if you remember that steroids are excellent short-term treatments for UC, and that the side effects are reduced by topical use, then it is surely worth considering.

Rectal steroids come in three forms:

- suppositories;
- liquid enemas; and
- foam enemas.

A suppository is a bullet-shaped tablet that is pressed into the rectum. The warmth of the body melts the suppository and the drug is gradually absorbed into the lining of the rectum. Suppositories are most suitable for proctitis because they do not travel into the colon. There may be an urge to force out the suppository, which should be resisted if possible.

People who have UC inflammation up the left side of the colon may consider using a liquid steroid enema such as Predenema® or Predsol®. This is because by lying in different positions it is possible to move the liquid enema up into the descending colon. The liquid enema consists of a bag containing the liquid steroid with a tube attached. The tube is inserted into the anus and the bag is slowly squeezed by hand so that the liquid enters the rectum in a steady stream. There may be some difficulty in avoiding leaks out of the anus, but this can usually be mastered with practice.

An alternative to a liquid enema is a foam enema (such as Predfoam® or Colifoam®). This is contained in a small pressurized container with an attached tube. The tube is inserted into the anus and one press of the button releases the necessary amount of steroid foam. The foam will not travel as far into the colon as the liquid enema, but it will stay in position more easily while the steroid is absorbed into the lining of the intestine.

Lynette
Early on I was prescribed steroid enemas. At first I found the idea of using them offensive. For most of us drug administration is orally, and any other way is indelicate to say the least. For me, they were of no use – I discharged them almost on contact, primarily because of the 'wind' I was plagued with. For the last 18 months, I have used suppositories, which I can retain for the necessary hour or so, lying on my left side. Again, I was apprehensive at the thought of using them, but you do get over that. They are easy to use provided you first scrape off the serrations left by the plastic wrapping!

For people whose UC inflammation covers a large part of their colon, systemic steroid tablets will be offered. These will also be offered to those patients who, for whatever reason, do not want a rectally administered drug. Taking medicines by mouth is very straightforward compared with enemas. Nevertheless it should be borne in mind that the side effects of corticosteroids are wide-ranging, and most people experience some problems when taking oral steroids. The main side effects are:

- weight-gain;
- swelling or rounding of the face;
- mood swings;
- acne;
- fluid retention leading to high blood pressure and swollen legs;
- sleeplessness;
- increased blood sugar level, with an increased risk of diabetes; and
- facial hair.

Barbara

My GP put me on a high dose of steroids and I quickly became manic. I would get up in the middle of the night to work and make sandwiches. I was always hungry and would have to eat huge amounts throughout the day. I swam like a dervish two or three times a week and would only feel relaxed when I took a steam bath after each swim.

Nicola

The steroids gave me some bad side effects – I put on weight (about a stone), my face really puffed up, I grew hair all over my arms and back and some on my face. It was horrible, but my bowel was getting better at last. I started reducing my steroids again, which I managed to do successfully this time ... It's now been eight months since I was first diagnosed with ulcerative colitis and six months since I was last in hospital. I'm now on other medication to keep the inflammation down, and my face has gone right back down to normal, the excess hair all came out and I feel a great deal better than when I was really ill.

If steroids are required for a long period, other side effects become important:

- softening of the bones;
- thinning of the muscles and skin, and a tendency to bruise easily; and
- eye problems such as cataracts or glaucoma.

Many of these side effects will recede when the amount of steroid is reduced or stopped altogether. Some of the side effects may become significant problems, however, if it becomes necessary to take steroids for a long period. If you are concerned about the possibility of bone thinning, ask your doctor for a bone density scan.

A new type of steroid drug, called budesonide (Entocort®), is a steroid that is taken by mouth and is released over a small area of the intestine. As such, smaller quantities enter the bloodstream, potentially reducing the level of side effects. Budesonide is designed for Crohn's disease, but it can be used in UC.

Stopping steroids

It is important to remember that when the symptoms of UC have been brought under control by the steroid drugs, the reduction in the amount of steroids must be undertaken slowly. It is very dangerous to stop taking steroids immediately. This is because the amount of natural hydrocortisone produced in the body will have reduced greatly during treatment because it was not needed. It takes time for the body to build up hydrocortisone production to its previous natural level. Therefore, if you reduce your steroid drugs suddenly, your body may struggle to cope with stressful situations.

Furthermore, during a traumatic accident, extra steroid production is needed to cope with the effects of shock. If you are taking steroids and your body's natural steroid production is not functioning, a steroid injection will be needed. If you are unconscious and are unable to tell a doctor that you regularly take steroid medication, no one will know to give the steroid injection and your body may fail to cope with the sudden demands placed on it. It is a good idea to carry a card, bracelet or necklace that gives information about your steroid drug regime. Your doctor should have information on the availability of these.

Barbara

I had a nasty experience when coming off steroids rather too abruptly. Driving home one morning, I felt I was going to pass out at the wheel. I managed to stop the car and phone for an ambulance. I made a swift recovery, but the experience taught me to treat steroids with more respect, and especially to reduce the dose very gradually.

Joanna

My illness gradually flared up again, and I found myself having to return to the hospital for more urgent appointments. It was then that they put me on my first course of oral steroids. What a wonder drug they were! Within a few days my flare-up had calmed down and I started to feel better. Although I knew the risk of osteoporosis in later life, I had felt so ill, that taking these 'wonder' tablets was well worth the risks – they were my lifeline. I am still taking the oral steroids, at a lower dose, as I know they will give me some relief from the illness. But my doctor at the hospital is keen for me to come off them completely, due to the risks, and for me to try an alternative drug.

In cases where it proves difficult to stop steroids altogether, without provoking a return of UC symptoms, doctors will look to other types of drugs to assist in keeping the disease under control.

Lynn
Having a supportive family and friends is a must. You can be a different person for a while when you are ill and on lots of medications, which can change your personality and certainly can affect your patience. Warning family and friends in advance is always useful.

Aminosalicylates

The drugs most commonly prescribed for maintaining remission from symptoms of UC are aminosalicylates, also known as 5-ASA. These drugs are related to aspirin, and they reduce inflammation. They will often be prescribed at the same time as steroids. Once the steroid drug has been stopped, the aminosalicylate drug will usually be continued in order to discourage a flare-up.

The potential for aminosalicylates to reduce UC was discovered in 1942. The first version of this drug was called sulphasalazine (Salazopyrin®). It had originally been developed as a treatment for rheumatoid arthritis. A patient with arthritis, who also had UC, was given sulphasalazine as a treatment for the arthritis. The unexpected result was that the UC improved substantially. Subsequently sulphasalazine became an established treatment for UC.

From the 1980s onwards, additional types of aminosalicylate were developed – mesalazine (Asacol®, Pentasa®, Salofalk®), olsalazine (Dipentum®) and balsalazide (Colazide®). All have a similar effect on UC, but some formulations work on slightly different parts of the intestine.

The main side effects of aminosalicylates are headache, nausea, diarrhoea and itchy skin. The newer drugs tend to have fewer side effects than sulphasalazine.

The range of choice of aminosalicylate drugs means that if you do not react well to one drug your doctor can usually find another type for you to try. These drugs are available in both oral and rectal form.

Barbara
Asacol® [mesalazine] certainly keeps my UC at bay but I believe it has annoying side effects. I often have headaches, feel nauseous and generally unwell, as if I am sickening for the flu. A good night's sleep usually puts things right.

Immunosuppressants

While steroids and aminosalicylates reduce inflammation, which is one process in the body's immune system, the third main category of drugs for UC works on the immune system as a whole. The immunosuppressant drugs were developed to counteract rejection of organ transplants. These drugs weaken the reaction of the immune system so that transplanted organs are more likely to be accepted. As UC involves the inappropriate reaction of the immune system, it was thought that drugs that suppress the response of immune cells might also reduce the severity of UC.

The two most commonly used immunosuppressants are azathioprine (Imuran®) and 6-mercaptopurine (Puri-Nethol®). These are both now accepted as effective treatments for UC. They are slow-acting drugs, often taking three months or more to have an effect on UC. They are very useful because of their 'steroid-sparing' effect. It is possible to reduce the amount of steroids taken if immunosuppressants are taken at the same time.

John
From 1975 to 2000 my treatment was based primarily on prednisolone, with some good periods but many not good. In November 2000 I started on azathioprine and reduced the prednisolone. I showed an amazing improvement.

The main drawback with immunosuppressant drugs is that they make people more vulnerable to infections, because a weakened immune system means that the body is in a poor position to defend itself from infectious bacteria and viruses. Therefore, if you are taking one of these drugs it is important to report to your doctor if you develop fever, chills or a persistent sore throat. Also, the number of white and red cells in the blood may be reduced, and so it is necessary to have regular blood tests.

The main side effects with azathioprine and 6-mercaptopurine are nausea, flu-like symptoms, abdominal pain and inflammation of the pancreas or liver. Up to 20 per cent of people taking azathioprine experience one or more of these side effects. Although 6-mercapto-purine is a similar drug, it may have fewer side effects.

Ciclosporin (Sandimmun®) is another immunosuppressant drug. It is used much less frequently than azathioprine and 6-mercaptopurine because its side effects are greater. Ciclosporin is mainly used for severe attacks, particularly if the UC is resistant to steroid treatment. In such cases it is usually given intravenously in hospital.

Heather
The consultant introduced oral steroids (prednisolone) to take with the sulphasalazine. The steroids were to be taken for a two-month period only (heavy dosage followed by gradual decline), which resulted in the following cycle: one month of getting better, one month of feeling well (by which time steroids have ended), followed by one month of niggling pain, then one month of vicious recurrence, followed by yet another course of steroids.

This cycle continued for about two years and then the consultant changed my medication to 400mg of mesalazine (Asacol®) three times a day and 50mg of azathioprine once a day, which finally did the trick! The azathioprine is commonly used by transplant patients to help prevent rejection of transplanted organs, but it works in combination with the mesalazine in combating my UC. I have to have regular liver function blood tests every two months as the azathioprine can possibly affect the liver, but so far all my blood tests have come back clear, no problems. Currently, I am in year two of remission, albeit with medication.

Other drugs

Reducing pain by using painkillers is problematic because a side effect of many painkillers is to disturb the digestive system. Non-steroidal anti-inflammatory drugs are a major category of painkillers, and include diclofenac (Voltarol®) and ibuprofen (Brufen®). All non-steroidal anti-inflammatory drugs should be avoided. The least troublesome painkiller is probably paracetamol.

Some drugs can reduce the symptoms of diarrhoea without affecting the level of inflammation. These antidiarrhoeal drugs, such as codeine phosphate (Kaodene®), loperamide (Imodium®) and diphenoxylate (Lomotil®), affect intestinal motility (muscle activity). By slowing the waves of movement of the intestine the contents move more slowly, providing more time for water to be absorbed into the body and for firmer stools to be formed. These anti-diarrhoeal drugs should not be taken on a regular basis, and they should definitely not be used in severe disease, because there is a risk of causing paralysis of the intestinal muscles, which in turn can lead to a dangerous condition called toxic dilatation (megacolon).

Constipation can be relieved by bulking agents (Fybogel®, Isogel®, Regulan®). By consuming these preparations with water, the fibre of the bulking agents fills out, making it easier for the intestine to move the contents along, and ending the constipation.

Antibiotics are normally only used in UC when the disease is very severe. A very inflamed intestine lets more bacteria pass into the bloodstream and there is a greater risk of developing infection. It is not uncommon for antibiotics to be prescribed as a preventative measure to patients who are in hospital for treatment of severe UC.

Blood loss in UC can lead to anaemia and it may become necessary to take iron supplements. These tablets darken the stool and may cause side effects of nausea, diarrhoea or constipation. Iron supplements are available as tablets, syrups or in an injectable form (for injection into a muscle or a vein). Long-term supplements of iron should be avoided, unless anaemia continues.

4

Diet

The small intestine, the part of the gut between the stomach and the colon, is concerned chiefly with digestion of food and the absorption of nutrients into the bloodstream. Enzymes are secreted into the small intestine to aid the breakdown of food particles into small molecules. The surface of the small intestine is covered by very large numbers of villi (tiny protrusions), which increase the surface area through which the nutrients can be absorbed into the body.

The colon, however, does not secrete digestive enzymes and it does not have villi. Furthermore, most nutrients have been removed by the time the contents of the intestine reaches the colon. It is argued, therefore, that the type of food that one eats has very little effect on or relevance to the state of a person's UC.

Nevertheless, information officers at the National Association for Colitis and Crohn's Disease report that a significant minority of people with UC who make telephone enquiries are adamant that changes in their diet have improved their symptoms.

Heather
I discovered that diet did affect my UC. Ordinary tea caused intense bloating and discomfort so I switched to herbal and fruit teas instead.

There is, therefore, some uncertainty over the role of diet in UC. This matter is considered more fully in this chapter under three headings – nutrition, fibre, and food intolerance.

Nutrition

If a body is well nourished by receiving a good quantity and variety of nutrients from digested food, then it is in a much better position to resist the effects of disease. This is as true for UC as it is for other diseases. People with UC can often be poorly nourished, becoming thin and feeling weak. It is important that they have a good balanced diet. The loss of weight and weakness may be caused by:

- reluctance to eat;
- loss of blood and mucus;
- anaemia;
- drugs that reduce the absorption of nutrients; and
- diarrhoea.

A reluctance to eat is understandable when a person knows that this may lead to diarrhoea and pain. Furthermore, someone who is feeling very unwell from the disease may simply lose his or her appetite. With insufficient calories, the body draws on fat reserves and the person becomes thinner. Being cautious about eating may also lead to the choice of a more limited range of foods, with an increased likelihood that some important vitamins or minerals may be missing.

The loss of blood and mucus from the intestinal wall, passed with the faeces, involves a loss of protein. This will need to be replaced, since protein is needed to repair the intestinal tissues. This repair demands energy, which may increase the feeling of weakness if insufficient calories are being consumed. Protein is also used for building muscles, and a loss of protein may lead to wasting muscles.

Anaemia is a shortage of haemoglobin in the blood. Haemoglobin is a protein that contains iron and is found in red blood cells. Haemoglobin carries oxygen from the lungs to tissues in all parts of the body. It also carries carbon dioxide away from tissues to the lungs. One of the ways in which anaemia develops is through heavy bleeding. Red blood cells are lost and along with them, haemoglobin. A decline in the capacity of blood to carry oxygen can cause fatigue, uncomfortable breathing, dizziness, headache, insomnia and pallor.

Some of the drugs used to treat UC can reduce the effectiveness of the intestine to absorb nutrients. For example, sulphasalazine (Salazopyrin®) may restrict the absorption of folic acid, and corticosteroids may change the way the body uses calcium, preventing it from strengthening bone.

Diarrhoea itself may cause weakness, because some nutrients and salts that would normally be absorbed into the body remain unabsorbed, owing to the rapid passage of the contents through the intestine.

If you are underweight or feeling weak, what should you do? First, discuss the matter with your doctor. The medical profession has traditionally focused on diagnosis and treatment rather than prevention. This has meant that the importance of good nutrition has been underplayed and has become mostly the responsibility of other health professionals such as nurses and dietitians. Do not assume that your doctor is uninterested in nutritional matters. He or she may refer you to a specialist nurse or a registered dietitian.

The nurse or dietitian will consider your medical history and discuss your concerns with you, possibly suggesting one or more of the following routes:

- reviewing your medications (in consultation with the doctor), with a view to bringing your disease under greater control. If the disease is in remission, you will feel more inclined to eat well, and your body will expend less energy coping with the effects of the disease;
- increasing the number of calories consumed. This can be achieved by introducing a greater variety of foods into your diet so that eating becomes more interesting. In general terms, for people with UC there are no particular foods that should be avoided. Another method of increasing calories is by eating smaller portions more often, such as six small meals a day;
- trying to eat a balanced diet. You may be given a guide to different types of food and the proportions that constitute an ideal balance;
- the addition of certain supplements, such as iron, calcium and folic acid (in consultation with the doctor), when there is likely to be a shortage not easily remedied by diet alone.

With the help of your health-care team, and the encouragement of your loved ones, it should be possible to feed your body well and build up your strength.

Fibre

Dietary fibre (also known as roughage) is a general term for the parts of food that are undigestible by enzymes in the mouth, stomach and small intestine. They are usually types of carbohydrate from plants. The amount and type of fibre in the diet is important for people with UC, because most of it reaches the colon unaltered and it influences both diarrhoea and constipation. In general terms, a high-fibre diet increases the likelihood of diarrhoea and a low-fibre diet carries the risk of constipation.

If a person has active UC with diarrhoea, it is sometimes recommended, in addition to taking drugs, that the amount of fibre in the diet is reduced. This should help reduce the diarrhoea, as more water will flow from the intestine into the body.

Maureen
A low-fibre diet was recommended. No fruit, restricted vegetables, no pork products, nothing fried. I followed this for years. I suffered constipation most of the time.

Once the diarrhoea has been brought under control, however, it is usually advisable not to continue a low-fibre diet, if possible. This is because dietary fibre has health benefits in other ways. For example, it reduces the amount of cholesterol in the blood and decreases the risk of developing haemorrhoids and diverticular disease. In people with UC it may not be easy to increase the amount of fibre in the diet without provoking the return of diarrhoea. There are, however, two main types of fibre, soluble and insoluble, and these have different effects on the intestine.

When soluble fibre is added to water, it produces a thick, sticky liquid that tends to be slow-moving. It is also fermentable by the bacteria in the colon, so that the mass of fibre is reduced as the faeces move forward. The reduction in mass tends to reduce any potential laxative effect that the soluble fibre may have at the end of the colon. Soluble fibre is also the type that reduces the level of cholesterol in the blood. In comparison, insoluble fibre may irritate the lining of the colon and accelerate the passage of the faeces through the colon, with a consequently greater risk of promoting diarrhoea. It would seem, therefore, that for people with UC soluble fibre may be more tolerable than insoluble fibre.

Some people with left-sided UC or proctitis develop constipation. Small hard stools are formed further up the colon from the area of inflammation, although it is not clear why this happens. The hard stools are not easily moved along the colon by peristalsis (muscular contractions) and tend to take longer than usual to reach the rectum. At this point they become difficult to pass through the anus, resulting in a lot of straining on the toilet.

Bulking agents may be prescribed to relieve the constipation. They have the effect of promoting regular and smooth peristalsis to move the content towards the rectum. Most of these bulk-forming products contain ispaghula, which is a form of soluble fibre.

Most plant foods contain both soluble and insoluble fibre. There are larger amounts of insoluble fibre in wholemeal bread, brown rice, bran, nuts, carrots, celery, tomatoes and fruits with edible seeds (such as raspberries). Larger quantities of soluble fibre are found in oats, barley, peas, beans, lentils, apples, citrus fruits, prunes and potatoes.

Each person is different but, in general terms, it is a good idea to obtain fibre from a broad range of foods, and to introduce any changes gradually. If you feel that altering the amount of fibre in your diet may help improve your symptoms, do speak with a specialist nurse or dietitian. Expert guidance is needed to identify the optimum level and type of fibre and the diet needed to achieve it.

Food allergy and intolerance

A small proportion of people with UC feel their condition is improved if they remove one or more foods from their diet. It is unlikely that a food allergy is present, since this affects only about 1 per cent of the general population and there is no evidence that there is a higher incidence of food allergy among people with UC. It is more likely that the reaction is a 'food intolerance'.

Definite statistics are not available on the prevalence of food intolerance, although it has been estimated to affect about 10 per cent of the general population. There is no evidence that food intolerance is more common among people with UC. The explanation for food intolerance is not known, but it is suspected that the particular food is either not fully digested owing to the shortage of an enzyme, or that the food contains a chemical that causes a reaction.

Heather
I have found, by bitter experience, that I don't suffer with UC attacks if I avoid:

- peanuts, mixed nuts, any nuts – I like them but they don't like me!;
- tea and coffee – doesn't matter if it's decaffeinated or not;
- bread, white, brown, wholemeal, toasted – intense bloating and discomfort follow;

- intensely spicy foods – goes without saying really!;
- rich fruit cake such as Christmas or wedding cake;
- dairy products (milk, yoghurts, ice cream, cream of any kind, and cheese);
- chocolate – if I indulge too much then my UC flares up, but I'm definitely not giving up chocolate (it's a woman thing!).

I rely on multi-vitamins and minerals (including iron and calcium) as well as cod-liver oil capsules to replace any nutrients that I'm unable to ingest.

Heather's list of foods is not intended as a recommended guide. Rather, it is included to show that some people with UC do benefit from avoiding certain foods. Each person is different and in most people with UC avoiding particular foods has no effect on intestinal disturbance.

Exclusion diets

The best way of checking for food intolerance is to undergo an exclusion diet (also known as an elimination diet), in which most types of food are removed from the diet to see if any symptoms are reduced. If there is no improvement, then it is concluded that the person's symptoms do not relate to food intolerance. If there is an improvement different foods are reintroduced gradually, one by one, to identify the ones that are causing the food intolerance.

If you want to check for food intolerance, it is important to discuss your wish with your doctor. There may be reasons why this may be a risky course of action. For example, you may be underweight and diet restrictions may be undesirable.

An exclusion diet developed by Dr John Hunter at Addenbrooke's Hospital, Cambridge, was tested on people with UC and on people with Crohn's disease. All normal foods were excluded and replaced by elemental diet, a special liquid drink consisting of sterile small molecules that provide balanced nutrition. The diet proved successful in producing remission in people with Crohn's disease, allowing the identification of troublesome foods by staged reintroductions. In people with UC, however, remission was not achieved as a result of the special diet.

This would suggest that food intolerance has little or no connection with UC. If a person has UC and coincidentally also has a food intolerance that is causing a digestive disturbance, the removal of that food from the diet will reduce the overall level of intestinal problems. It seems unlikely, however, that its removal will affect the level of inflammation caused by UC.

Dr Hunter's exclusion diet (described in his book *The New Allergy Diet* – see Further reading on page 104) is initially quite drastic in removing so many types of food, and is therefore usually undertaken under medical supervision.

An alternative is Brostoff and Gamlin's elimination diet. This diet involves a three-stage process and reduces the likelihood of having to give up foods unnecessarily. Details may be found in their book *The Complete Guide to Food Allergy and Intolerance* (see Further reading on page 104).

Lactose intolerance

One of the best-known examples of food intolerance is lactose intolerance. Lactose is a sugar found in dairy products and is sometimes referred to as 'milk sugar'. The enzyme in the small intestine that digests lactose is called lact*ase*. Lactase breaks the lactose into two simpler sugars that are easily absorbed through the intestine into the bloodstream. People who are lactose-intolerant do not produce enough of the enzyme lactase to digest all the milk sugar consumed, and some of the lactose moves unaltered towards the lower part of the intestine. The undigested lactose draws water into the intestine and this may lead to cramping pain as the gut muscles strain ineffectively to move the liquid contents. Diarrhoea may also develop. In the colon, the resident bacteria ferment the lactose and produce lots of gas that causes bloating, pain and flatus (passing of wind).

If you find that you are lactose-intolerant, in addition to avoiding dairy products, it is also worth checking the ingredients of processed foods. Lactose is used by the food industry as a cheap filler and is also part of several food ingredients – casein, caseinate, sodium caseinate, whey, lactoglobulin, lactalbumen and curds.

The permanent removal of milk, butter, cheese and similar foods from the diet has some nutritional disadvantages. In particular, it may cause a shortage of calcium. This is an important matter for people taking corticosteroids and for older women. Steroids weaken bones if taken for a long time, and older women are at a higher risk of developing osteoporosis as a result of the hormonal changes that occur after menopause. Calcium supplements may be recommended

if there are signs of bone thinning, although care must be taken not
to exceed the dose since this may promote constipation.

If you have to remove most dairy products from your diet, try
yoghurt and mature hard cheese to see if they prove tolerable. The
bacteria added to these foods produce the enzyme lactase themselves, and this helps to digest the lactose.

Steve

I have to consider everything I put into my mouth – will this
cause embarrassing stomach eruptions or drastically affect output
consistency? I'm often told that eating this or that food or drink
will not do me any good, but I must admit that my prime
consideration is 'how will it affect my stomach?' not 'is this good
for me?'. I often decline the most mouth-watering temptations (to
the surprise of any company) for fear of the effect they may have.
The type of food or drink probably makes no difference when the
colitis is at this advanced stage and I believe the daily variations
in stomach activity would be just as volatile regardless of what I
ate or drank provided it was in moderation.

Christine

I have never associated my flare-ups to anything I have eaten.

Joanne

I have looked at various changes in diet, but excluding certain
foods really doesn't benefit me at all. The only foods that seem to
make my UC much worse are custard-based products. However,
cream cakes I'm OK with, so I'm grateful for that!

In the complicated area of food allergy and intolerance it is
important to work closely with your doctor and to avoid people with
dubious qualifications. Otherwise you may be persuaded to remove
foods from your diet unnecessarily and risk reducing your nutrition.

5

Living with ulcerative colitis

Once you have been diagnosed with UC, a wide range of feelings and practical issues may arise.

Adjusting to a long-term condition

There may be immediate concerns about taking medications and bringing the disease under control. Some time later, however, your attention may switch to thinking about having a disease for which there is currently no cure and that may cause you difficulties for the rest of your life.

This realization can be a shock. It may lead to a range of reactions, including:

- emotional denial that the disease exists;
- anger that your life may be seriously affected through no fault of your own;
- a sense that you have less control over your life;
- a fear that the illness will make others not love or respect you;
- a period of depression.

Whatever your reaction, you will have your own way of coping. Three commonly used methods are:

- carrying on with life as if nothing has changed;
- talking with friends and loved ones; and
- learning everything possible about the disease.

You may have a different approach, or a combination of those listed above. Whatever your preferred method of coping, do consider whether this method is a positive choice rather than just the usual way you deal with difficulties. The difference here is that UC is likely to be with you for a long time (unless you have major surgery). A successful coping strategy for the long term may need more conscious thought.

If you carry on as if nothing has changed, others may admire your stoicism and treat you with increased respect. You will also have the comforting thought that you are not being a burden on others. However, people may underestimate the degree to which UC can disrupt your life (for instance, that you may need to plan outings around the availability of toilets). Also, over time, the demands of the illness may become overwhelming. It may be difficult for you to acknowledge this if you are used to the 'I can cope' strategy. To reduce the risk of such a 'breakdown' if things become too much for you, it might be worth considering using other strategies as well.

You may, for example, find that talking to someone is helpful. Is your reluctance to talk about your worries because you have had very little practice of doing so in the past? Or is it because you fear that the person you speak to may have less respect for you? There is much to be said for the stoical approach, but do make sure that you adopt it because it suits your personality and beliefs, rather than because it is the only approach you know.

Joanne

A lot of people I work with have said they would never have guessed I have UC if I hadn't told them. I suppose the only visible sign is when I lose a noticeable amount of weight, as I have at the moment. People ask me if I'm dieting – I wish I was!

I find it really helps to talk to people about my illness. I have a lot of supportive friends and am lucky to have a neighbour who also suffers with UC, which has been a big help.

For those who enjoy talking with their friends, the benefits of conversation are patently obvious. Worries that can buzz around inside the head, making one anxious and perhaps feeling 'a little mad', can dissipate with a sympathetic heart-to-heart talk. Having someone acknowledge that you are distressed and that your worries are not unreasonable can be comforting. Also, by sharing your personal concerns you are indirectly telling the listener that he or she is important to you and is needed, which is a comfort to the person concerned. There are disadvantages to this approach, however. Firstly, it may be difficult to find friends who are willing to listen to you and discuss bowel problems. Also, if you talk too much about your illness and its consequences, you may place too much of a burden on your friend and threaten your friendship. There is also the risk that talking about a problem can sometimes be an alternative to doing something about it. You might wish to consider whether you can carry more of the burden yourself and learn more about the disease so that there are fewer unknowns to make you anxious.

The third main strategy, of learning about the condition, has the advantage that you may be reassured that there is no imminent 'breakthrough' treatment of which you are unaware. Also, in knowing about the disease you will be able to speak more confidently with your doctor. This can be particularly useful if you are having trouble with your medication and want to talk about possible changes, or if a major decision such as surgery has to be made. Furthermore, if there are alternative therapies that look promising, you can investigate and discuss them with your doctor. The disadvantage with the learning strategy is that it can sometimes be used as an excuse for not facing up to the day-to-day problems caused by the disease. By desperately holding out for a cure, you may delay the process of accepting the condition and adapting to it.

Nicola
When I first found out that I had ulcerative colitis, I did think 'I'm only 19 years old, what have I done to deserve a long-term illness?' But you just have to accept it and get on with life. It's no good sitting and feeling sorry for yourself all the time.

If adjusting to this long-term condition is proving difficult, you could discuss with your doctor whether there are any psychological or counselling services available that may help you. If you are religious, do not forget about prayer.

Long-term worries

Whatever strategy you use for coping with UC, there may still be underlying worries that continue. A survey of opinion among people with UC found that the most frequently mentioned worries were:

- uncertainty about the future;
- side effects of medication;
- lack of energy;
- the need for an ileostomy; and
- the development of colon cancer.

Uncertainty about the future

One of the difficulties with UC is that it fluctuates from flare-up to remission. You do not know how long either period will last. It may be necessary to adopt a more philosophical attitude, so that you do not worry all the time about what will happen next. This is, of course, easier said than done.

Jean

It was when I started a job that my UC ceased to be first and foremost to me. I had doubts as to whether I could maintain a job if I had to keep going to the loo, but it has worked out. I would strongly recommend people getting involved with other interests, be it a job, charity work, learning a hobby or yoga. Ideally, do something to take you out of the house and mix with other people ... It is such a confidence boost to realize that you can do it and you begin to realize that UC is not going to dominate your life.

Even when you are feeling well, there may be a nagging fear that you will suddenly have a desperately urgent need to go to the toilet. One way of dealing with this problem is to imagine the most embarrassing and humiliating consequences of having an 'accident' in public. How would you cope? Thinking about this might help you to accept that the embarrassing situations you most fear can in fact be managed and that you do not have to turn yourself into a recluse.

Liz

I try to keep a sense of humour. At one time, I was experiencing a lot of very unpleasant flatulence and got to the front of a queue in a shop as people moved out of the way!

Side effects of medication

Many people with UC need to take prescribed drugs for the rest of their lives. The drugs used to control UC are quite strong and side effects can occur.

Corticosteroids are the type of drug most effective in bringing the inflammation of UC under control. They also cause the most side effects (as described in Chapter 3). The effect on appearance can be particularly distressing for teenagers and young adults, and mood swings can make life difficult for family members. Remember, though, if you want to come off steroids these drugs cannot be reduced quickly, because the body's natural steroids need time to increase. Slow reduction is also desirable because a relapse is less likely to be triggered.

The aminosalicylate drugs can also have side effects and it is important to consider alternatives. For people with UC, if sulphasalazine (Salazopyrin®) is not well tolerated, there are several mesalazine products that can be considered, as well as olsalazine (Dipentum®) and balsalazide (Colazide®).

Lack of energy

The cause of lethargy in people with UC is not fully understood. It may be due to a number of factors:

- undernourishment, caused by a lack of appetite;
- loss of protein from the inflamed colon;
- loss of blood, resulting in anaemia;
- sleeplessness arising from nocturnal diarrhoea;
- a result of the inflammatory process itself.

Joanne

As I'm still in and out of bed at night with my UC, I've adjusted my sleep pattern, particularly when I'm at work in the week. I go to bed earlier to try and compensate for the times I'm up in the early hours. If I feel tired when I come home from work (which is most days!), I try and catch half an hour's nap on the settee before my tea (if my UC lets me) and I find that helps as well.

The decrease in energy that can accompany UC may profoundly affect how you see yourself. You may fear that your health will gradually deteriorate to the point that the disease has a disabling effect on your daily life. It does not necessarily follow, however, that if you are feeling unwell and weak now that further deterioration is inevitable. UC is a fluctuating condition and it can improve. Also, new and better treatments are continually appearing.

Do not be afraid to seek help from your family and friends when you are feeling fatigued. Some people confuse tiredness with laziness so it is important that you describe how you feel.

Lynette

I live alone and have often thought this to be fortunate because UC is definitely a most unsociable disease! However, with UC one can become very debilitated with weight loss, energy loss, loss of appetite, etc. At these times, when you are so unwell that even to make a cup of tea is akin to climbing Everest, family around you would be welcome.

You may be concerned about the economic effect of not being as dynamic an employee as you have been in the past. The lethargic feeling is associated with active disease, however, and once the UC has been brought under control, fresh energy is likely to develop. Take advantage of periods of remission to build up your strength by eating well and by taking regular exercise. It may also be worthwhile to review your career plans and consider whether your current type of work is really what you want or whether it is sustainable with a fluctuating illness. If you fear that you may be dismissed while being temporarily unable to work, consider seeking legal advice on your employment rights, including eligibility for protection under the Disability Discrimination Act.

The need for an ileostomy

The thought of having an ileostomy, a piece of intestine protruding out of your abdomen, can be repugnant. For some people the determination to avoid this alteration to their body's appearance dominates their thinking about UC. They have a major incentive to take all medications exactly as prescribed, and to explore all other routes to reduce symptoms.

For some people with UC, however, no matter how hard they try to improve the situation, the inflammation of their colon is very severe and their quality of life is very poor. In those cases, as is explained in Chapter 7, a total colectomy is required, involving the surgical removal of the whole colon. This is a major operation, but it has been undertaken so often by surgeons that it is now considered routine. A scar on the abdomen is left. Once it has healed, the scar does not usually cause great concern, although some women decide that they will wear one-piece swimming costumes instead of bikinis.

An important issue for people who are due to have a colectomy is how the faeces will be excreted. An ileostomy used to be the only option, but now there is the alternative possibility of an internal pouch formed from the end of the small intestine. The internal pouch is attached to the rectum, so that faecal matter can still be passed through the anus.

Both an ileostomy and an internal pouch have their advantages and disadvantages, which are discussed in Chapter 8. It does not automatically follow that an internal pouch is better for a person than an ileostomy, nor is an internal pouch achievable in all people with UC who are to have a colectomy.

If an ileostomy has to be formed, a consoling thought, for people who dread it, is that they are likely to feel immensely better (because there is no longer any UC). Also, over a period of time, most people get used to having a stoma.

Development of colon cancer

Of all long-term worries for people with UC, fear of developing colon cancer is usually the greatest. This is, of course, because there is a fairly high mortality rate with colon cancer.

It should be noted that people with proctitis (UC affecting the rectum only) or proctosigmoiditis (UC affecting the rectum and the sigmoid colon) do not appear to have any increased risk of cancer over the general population. This does not mean that they cannot develop it, but rather that there is no extra risk as a consequence of having inflammation just of the rectum or sigmoid colon. For people with extensive UC or pancolitis (UC covering most or all of the colon) there is an increased risk of developing cancer in the colon or rectum after about eight years with UC. The statistics on the level of risk are not very clear, but a recent review of available data concluded that:

- after 20 years of UC, 5–10 per cent will develop colorectal cancer;
- after 25 years of UC, approximately 15 per cent will develop colorectal cancer;
- after 35 years of UC, up to 30 per cent will develop colorectal cancer.

Statistics for people with left-sided UC are not reliable. It is suspected that there is an increased risk, although not as great as for people with pancolitis.

If you come from a family that has a history of colon cancer, then your risk of developing it may be higher, since genetic factors are also involved. By being aware of how extensive your UC is and also of any family history of colon cancer, you will get a better picture of your level of risk.

The best way to monitor the risk is by having regular colonoscopies. The frequency of such examinations varies from hospital to hospital. One approach is to have a colonoscopy every two to three years for people with left-sided UC, extensive UC or pancolitis that has been present for more than seven years. This surveillance may be increased to once a year for those who have had this degree of UC for more than 15 years.

Signs of cancer can be identified by taking biopsies (small samples) from the wall of the colon during a colonoscopy and examining them in the laboratory. There is a new technique that entails spraying the colon with a dye to help identify pre-cancerous signs and therefore the best places to take biopsies. If there is any doubt as to whether a colonoscopy has identified early signs of cancer, a total colectomy is usually recommended as a protective measure. This subject is discussed further in Chapter 7.

If you appear to be at significant risk, you can ask your doctor to arrange for more frequent colonoscopies. In this way you can keep this major fear under more reasonable control.

Personal relationships

Those who love you will react in various ways to your illness. And your illness may influence the way in which you react to your loved ones.

If you are still living with your parents, there is sometimes a tendency for them to be overprotective. Their love for you may make them feel very upset when you are unwell. As there may be times when you cannot look after yourself very well, your incapacity may bring back patterns of behaviour that your parents used when you were a child and were more dependent upon them. Try to be understanding about them wanting to help, but if their help becomes too claustrophobic or undermines your ability to be independent, it may be sensible to let them know this, gently.

If you have children, they may have difficulties in accepting your being unwell. They may expect their parents to be strong and reliable all the time, and it may be unsettling to find you otherwise.

Some young children might blame themselves, because they may have had angry thoughts about you in the past. Also, children may be disappointed if you cannot participate in family outings and school events. It is not unnatural to feel guilty about missed activities, but if you are not well enough it is not your fault; try to compensate with activities that you *are* capable of doing with them. Children can become more mature when they learn that not everyone is strong all the time and that each of us requires help in certain situations.

Close family members can play an important role in providing support and encouragement, but they need to understand the condition in the first place.

Rita
The worst part is the urgency – you don't get any warning. You have to go there and then and you can still have accidents even in your own home, so you tend to become a bit of a recluse. I know I have missed out on such a lot of events, such as with the grandchildren, holidays and trips out. I have to really make a big effort to go and do the weekly shop, often having to abandon my trolley in the middle of the shop and do a runner. But now I have got my husband to help. In the early stages of the illness, I don't think the family could understand what was the matter. I joined the NACC [National Association for Colitis and Crohn's Disease] and got quite a bit of information from them, but it wasn't until my eldest and youngest daughters went with me to a meeting, where my doctor was giving a talk, that they fully understood what I was going through.

Other family members, particularly those who know you less well and who know less about UC, may have simplistic ideas about the condition. Possible reactions are:

- if you ate a healthy balanced diet you wouldn't have this problem;
- everyone has diarrhoea every now and then, so why make such a fuss?;
- if you weren't so stressed the intestines would settle down;
- you would do better to get plenty of exercise, instead of resting so much.

You can try to explain about UC and give them leaflets, but you may also have to accept that not everyone has the time, patience or sympathy to take in new information. They may have worries of their own.

You may find considerable support and sympathy among your friends, but it may not necessarily be easy for them to understand a disease that shows few external signs, and yet never quite goes away. On the other hand, having a long-term illness means that those people who continue to be your friends are likely to be good and true friends. Do not forget that friendship is a two-way process and that being ill is not an excuse to avoid putting effort into maintaining and developing friendships. If you find, despite your best efforts, that you have very few friends, you could consider joining NACC (see Sources of help, page 101) and becoming an active member of the local group. Alternatively, you could join a club or hobby group on a subject that interests you and that is completely unconnected to bowel disease. Forgetting about UC for a while can be very refreshing.

If you are unmarried or do not have a long-term partner, having UC can lead to considerable anxiety about whether you will meet someone who will fall in love with you. The symptoms of UC may affect your confidence and how attractive you feel. It is important to remember that all of us have our strengths and weaknesses, and a potential spouse will love you as a whole person. If your UC is making you reluctant to socialize, however, you may need to make a conscious effort to meet people. Showing an interest in other people, and not worrying too much about your problems, is likely to make you more attractive.

In a marriage, the development of a chronic condition like UC can put a great deal of strain on the relationship. The person with UC might have reduced career opportunities, with financial consequences, or may not be able to contribute much to the housework. Sexual relations may also become more inhibited and less frequent. These stresses and strains may break up the marriage or, alternatively, make it stronger. The difference might be the couple's willingness to approach problems that arise, honestly and openly.

In particular, sexual relations may be affected by fears about incontinence (leaking from the bowel) and by a feeling of tiredness or pain. If you undergo surgery it may take several months before you feel strong enough or confident enough to engage in sexual

45

intercourse. Please remember, however, that sexual love can be expressed by holding and caressing as well as by intercourse and that it is often the feelings behind the expression of sexual love that are as important as the physical acts. Being able to talk with your partner about sexual worries may not come easily, but it is a good idea to do this to stop a barrier to intimacy undermining the relationship.

Coping with diarrhoea

Brenda
At parties I was on edge all the time. I was worried that someone else would be using the loo when I needed to go. I became a bit of a hermit.

One of the most inhibiting aspects of UC is diarrhoea, which can be very hard to control. Fear of having an 'accident' may dominate daily life. There are a number of practical steps that can be undertaken to relax the grip of this fear.

Take an emergency kit (such as spare underwear, moist wipes, panty liners if you are worried about leaks, and deodorizer) wherever you go. Then, if the worst occurs and you soil yourself, you are at least in a better position to deal with the consequences.

Obtain a RADAR key (see Sources of help, page 101) for disabled toilets. This is very useful when you need to be in a toilet cubicle, especially if you need to clean some of your clothing. Carrying a 'can't wait' card is also useful and reassuring, if you might need to use staff toilets in a shopping centre. This card explains that you have urgent need of a toilet as the result of a non-infectious condition and is available from NACC, CICRA (Crohn's in Childhood Research Association) or the Continence Foundation (see Sources of help, page 100).

Clair
All pubs have toilets and most big shops, as well as 99 per cent of cafés. If you have to buy a drink you don't need to drink it! I have never used my 'can't wait' card; I'd be too mortified. I just ask if I can use their loo and have never in 17 years been refused. When I go to the cinema or theatre I always sit in an aisle seat. It is easier to get in and out for the loo should I need to. I always carry a toilet bag with me. In it I have a small packet of baby wipes, a

pack of tissues and a spare pair of pants. I drive regularly to see my Mum, over an hour away. In my car I have an old track suit, and if I have an accident I can always get changed. These little things have made all the difference between missing out on life or going prepared and living a little.

The urge to have a bowel motion is often at its strongest soon after consuming a meal. This is caused by the gastrocolic reflex, which is an automatic response of the body in which strong muscle contractions of the colon push faeces towards the rectum, with resulting pressure to pass stools. This urge to have a bowel motion is at its strongest about 30 minutes after completing a meal. In most people this urge can be controlled; however, in some people with UC it may be uncontrollable. If the gastrocolic reflex tends to have a powerful effect on you, you may need to plan to be within easy reach of a toilet half an hour after eating a meal away from home.

If you have to go to the toilet many times a day, the area around your anus may become tender or sore. Occasionally an anal fissure may develop, which is a cut or tear of the skin near the anus. This may be very painful during a bowel motion. In order to soothe the area and avoid infection, both for anal soreness and for anal fissures, bathe your bottom in warm water in a large bowl (or use a bidet). Adding salt to the water can help reduce any infection. Clean the area with cotton wool and dry with very soft toilet paper. Your doctor or nurse may recommend an ointment to protect the skin.

Sarah
A raised toilet seat was an invaluable aid to me during my fissure episode. It enabled me not to have to lower myself down on to the toilet, which would stretch the anal area and cause further irritation. Aids such as these are usually available on free loan through the GP.

If you are leaking from your anus, one explanation is that your anal sphincter muscles are not strong. It may be worth trying pelvic floor exercises, instructions for which should be available from your doctor or nurse.

Craig
I started a home wine- and beer-making retail business and for the first 18 months I worked alone. With increasing frequency I would have to lock my shop door and dash to the toilet to relieve

myself, and wash and change if I had had an accident. I was always determined not to give up trying to follow a normal life, but wherever I went the first thing I had to do was locate the toilets. Often when travelling in my car I would have to stop and jump over a nearby hedgerow (thank goodness I live in a rural community) to relieve myself.

Travel

For most people with UC, there should be no reason why they cannot go away on holiday. Some thought and preparation may be needed beforehand, however.

Susan
When we go on holiday abroad, we only go for a week or 10 days. I can feel my colitis starting to flare up due to the change in water and food, even though I drink bottled water and am so careful what I eat. I still enjoy myself, though.

Here is a list of points you may need to think about when travelling on holiday, especially abroad:

- take a letter from your doctor describing your condition and listing the medications that you take (your doctor may make a charge for this);
- take more of the medications than you need for the holiday period and keep them in separate bags in case you lose some of them;
- make sure that you have travel insurance that covers pre-existing conditions so that you can be reimbursed if you have medical or hospital expenses associated with your UC;
- if travelling to a European Union country, acquire a stamped E111 form that will entitle you to free or reduced-cost State-provided emergency treatment;
- ask to sit near a toilet on the aircraft.

Julia
I started skiing when I was 30, a couple of years after having my UC diagnosed. Skiers are up and out on the mountain as soon as the lifts open at 9 a.m. Not a good time for me. There was nothing

more frustrating than getting on your ski boots, gloves etc, and then getting the warning signals of an imminent need for the loo. Thank goodness for codeine phosphate. Ski lessons are also usually first thing in the morning and last two hours. It is very difficult to try to explain to a French ski instructor that you may need to stop for the loo briefly during the lesson. Because of this I somehow always managed to hold on.

One of my main problems with skiing was the outer clothing, especially the trousers or salopettes. Your ski jacket goes over the top of the trousers so there is no quick and easy removal of your lower clothing, especially as you have thick gloves on too. I was usually found shedding various items of clothing and leaving a trail of them en route to the loo. One good thing are ski boots as you can get into a good squatting position over an undesirable loo by leaning into the boots as they give good support!

I was always able to ski very fast down a mountain when I needed the loo. There is nothing like desperation to drastically improve your skiing ability, albeit temporarily!

If you are visiting friends and are concerned about the possibility of night-time incontinence, you could take your own spare towels to be laid on the bed. You could also take a plastic potty for the bedroom so that you do not have to search for a strange bathroom in a hurry.

Caroline
When staying at a friend's home I had to go to the toilet urgently at night. I didn't make it and had an accident – on a white carpet! It was almost unbearable having to explain to my friend. It isn't always possible to avoid these accidents, so now I explain about my UC to any friends I'm visiting, saying something like, 'It can make me rather incontinent – and I don't mean just pee. I just can't get to a loo in time.' That's a way of saying something quite clearly without spelling it out.

6

Non-intestinal complications

For some people, UC is associated with complications in other parts of the body apart from the intestines. The affected parts can include:

- the joints;
- the skin;
- the mouth;
- the eyes;
- the liver and kidneys;
- the veins; and
- the bones.

Some of these complications are closely associated with a flare-up of the UC, but others are not.

Joints

Between 10 and 20 per cent of people with UC are affected by inflammation of the joints, such as the knees, ankles, elbows and wrists. The inflammation can take the form of arthralgia, a relatively mild aching of the joints. Arthritis may also develop, with the joint being red and swollen and movement becoming restricted. There may be severe pain. The good news is that the joint inflammation rarely leads to any permanent damage, and it will usually disappear when the intestinal inflammation has been brought under control.

Often, only one joint is affected, although sometimes several joints become inflamed. Inflammation sometimes moves from one joint to another. Less commonly, the small joints, in toes and fingers, are affected.

In hard-to-treat cases of UC-related arthritis, steroid injections into the affected joint can be given. It is also important to keep joints moving with a little exercise to avoid them getting very stiff.

Between 5 and 10 per cent of people with UC have inflammation of spinal joints. This can take the form of sacroiliitis, in which a joint (the sacroiliac joint) in the lower back is inflamed, leading to pain and morning stiffness. As lower back stiffness and pain is a common ailment, it is not always easy to diagnose sacroiliitis. It often precedes a flare-up of UC by days or weeks. Medications used to reduce inflammation of the colon also work on this lower back inflammation.

A more serious form of spine inflammation is ankylosing spondylitis. This affects the joints of the spine, causing pain and stiffness. In severe cases the spine can become rigid. It is diagnosed by X-ray. About 5 per cent of people with UC are affected. The development of ankylosing spondylitis tends to occur independently of UC, although the two diseases are associated. Treatment includes vigorous physiotherapy and sleeping on a hard bed.

The difficulty with joint inflammations is that the most effective painkillers, the non-steroidal anti-inflammatory drugs, also cause intestinal disturbance, so pain control is difficult.

Skin

Two main types of skin disease affect people with UC. Erythema nodosum causes tender red nodules below the skin, particularly on the lower part of the legs. These nodules last for several days or weeks and leave a brownish skin colouration. Erythema nodosum is usually associated with a flare-up of colitis and ceases when the UC goes into remission. About 8 per cent of people with UC develop erythema nodosum. It is most common in younger women.

Pyoderma gangrenosum is a more serious but less common condition that affects about 2 per cent of people with UC. It causes pustules (pus-filled blisters) on the skin, usually the legs, which develop into blue–red ulcers. These ulcers are not usually painful, but they are unsightly and hard to treat. They may need dressings to avoid infection. Usually pyoderma gangrenosum heals over time, but occasionally skin grafts are needed. As with erythema nodosum, the cause is not known. Unlike erythema nodosum, pyoderma gangrenosum is often not directly associated with UC flare-ups.

Eyes

Less than 5 per cent of people with UC are affected by inflammation of the eyes. There are two types, the first being episcleritis. This affects the white of the eye and causes the blood vessels to become dilated. The eyes burn and itch, and there is increased tear production. Sometimes the area around the eyelashes reddens. Although episcleritis is an irritating condition, it is not serious and usually ceases as the UC goes into remission.

The second type of eye inflammation associated with UC is uveitis (also known as iritis), in which the coloured part of the eye, the iris, is affected. The symptoms are pain in the eyes, blurred vision, increased sensitivity to light and, sometimes, headaches. It is mostly men who are affected. If untreated, permanent damage to the eye may occur, so it is important to see an ophthalmologist.

Both types of eye inflammation can be treated with steroid eye drops.

Liz

I still don't know if it was just coincidence or related in some way, but at the same time as the severe UC symptoms, my lower back 'locked' and I was in constant, extreme pain. I had to borrow a wheelchair from a friend just to get about the house. I also developed white spots on the edge of my eyelids, making my vision blurry and also causing dozens of mouth ulcers. I had not eaten much food for some time, but with the ulcers I could hardly drink water.

Mouth

Clusters of mouth ulcers occasionally appear at times of active UC. They usually last for a week or two. Less than 5 per cent of people with UC are affected.

Liver and kidneys

In about 5 per cent of people with UC, the bile ducts (which carry digestive juices from the liver to the gut) become inflamed, hardened and narrowed. This condition is known as primary sclerosing cholangitis, and it causes symptoms of abdominal pain, fever, chills, fatigue, itching of the skin and jaundice. It affects more men than women, and it is diagnosed by blood tests or magnetic resonance imaging. Its cause is not known. Treatment of primary sclerosing cholangitis is not very effective. Over time the liver may become severely damaged and eventually a liver transplant may be needed.

There is a risk of developing kidney stones with UC if you are prone to dehydration. Stones can cause excruciatingly sharp pain, but most stones are passed in the urine without special treatment.

Veins

In up to 5 per cent of people with UC, vein walls become inflamed, particularly in the legs. The inflammation leads to a thickening of blood and the development of thromboses (blood clots). Symptoms vary, depending on the deepness of the affected veins. Limbs may become pale, cool, swollen, itchy, aching and sensitive to pressure.

There is a risk that one of the blood clots may travel through the bloodstream and lodge in the lungs, as a pulmonary embolus. This is very dangerous and can be fatal. Treatment involves the use of anti-clotting drugs, such as heparin and warfarin, neither of which worsens UC.

Steve

My leg was so painful I visited the doctor twice, initially being told that the pain was to be expected if I played squash and football regularly. I was then hospitalized, with blood clots on the lung (pulmonary emboli) being diagnosed. The clots were dissolved (using heparin) and the colitis brought into remission with intravenous steroids and enemas. A year later, I was readmitted with more clots on the lung and after a similar drug blast I was released, but now have to take warfarin on a daily basis.

The development of emboli is more likely in people who are bed-ridden or dehydrated. If you cannot leave your bed, move your body regularly by wriggling your toes, bending your knees and generally moving your limbs. This will help to move blood through the veins. If you are more mobile, try to walk as much as possible. Make sure you drink plenty of fluids.

Bones

People with UC are more prone to bone thinning. It is known that this is caused by corticosteroids, but it may also be that the inflammatory process itself contributes to the thinning. Elderly people and post-menopausal women are at higher risk, as are those who live a sedentary life.

There are few clear signs of osteoporosis, but lower back pain, loss of height and fractures of the backbone, hips and wrists are all indications that it is present. There is a bone densitometry test that can indicate whether bones are thin. The equipment is available in hospitals.

Calcium and vitamin D are needed to increase bone strength. Calcium is readily available in milk and dairy products, and vitamin D can be generated through sunshine on the skin, or through consuming oily fish. Calcium supplements and fish liver oil can be taken if necessary. Hormone replacement therapy may be helpful for post-menopausal women, although there are some risks associated with this treatment, which your doctor can explain. Avoid being overweight and take regular exercise to promote bone development and improve flexibility. Bisphosphonates are a new type of drug that may also help reduce osteoporosis. If you are at high risk of bone weakness, do discuss with your doctor the options open to you.

7
Surgery

The proportion of people with UC who are obliged to have their colon removed at some time in their life is somewhere between one-fifth and one-third. It is not possible to be more precise about this, because there are no universally accepted statistics as to the total number of people with UC. It is clear, however, that those who do have surgery are a minority. It is also known that the larger the area of the colon affected by UC, the more likely it is that surgery will be required.

Most people with UC who have surgery have made a careful and conscious choice about the matter. This is known by doctors as 'elective' surgery. The main reasons for choosing a colectomy (removal of the colon) are:

- continuing deterioration in quality of life; and
- risk of developing cancer of the colon.

Quality of life

For some people, UC is brought under control by drugs and they have long periods of time when the disease is in remission. For others, symptoms never really go away, despite high levels of medication. Furthermore, the more severe the UC, the more likely a person will have symptoms in other parts of the body (for example, arthritis-like pain or inflammation of the eyes – see Chapter 6).

With any long-term illness, the general health can decline gradually. You may become cautious about leaving home without plotting where the public toilets are, you may take less exercise for fear of an 'accident', your work and social opportunities may become restricted, and you may gradually become more lethargic. Sometimes it is hard to notice how much your activities have become limited – it is easier for friends to notice the deterioration. A time may come when your doctor feels little more can be done to help through drugs and that surgery is therefore the best option.

Sam
The UC returned with venom. I tried to hide its impact, but I grew weaker and weaker. Often I would spend an hour lying on the

bathroom floor after fainting. The pain was intense, I was losing large amounts of blood and had become anaemic . . . Seven years on from the first attack of UC, they have decided to operate and at last remove the bowel. My little girl is thrilled, she knows that her Mum is going to have a 'magic bag' – which will mean that her Mum can do things she has never been able to do with her before.

Many people resist this suggestion with great determination. If one is young, then to have the permanent removal of a substantial part of one's innards can seem unnecessarily drastic. If one is older, there may be anxiety about the risks of any operation, or a reluctance 'to give up now' after surviving so long without an operation.

However, many people with UC on having had a colectomy say that they wish they had had the operation sooner. They feel so much better, experiencing no diarrhoea or pain and regaining energy. Many feel they have started a new life.

Cancer of the colon

The second reason for elective surgery is when a colonoscopy has found abnormal signs in the colon, which might be an early indication of cancer. The signs can be dysplasia, which are abnormal cells shown under the microscope from a biopsy taken from the mucosa (lining of the colon), or polyps (lumps or protrusions) on the colon wall, visible by the colonoscope camera.

If dysplasia or polyps are found, it does not mean that cancer has developed. Doctors do, however, use these signs as an indication that they should recommend a colectomy. The patient can then decide. It is not possible to predict whether cancer will develop, although it is known that the larger the area of colon affected by UC and the longer a person has had UC, the higher the risk of cancer.

When advised that a colonoscopy has shown abnormalities in the colon, most people decide to have their colon removed as a safety precaution, because cancer of the colon carries with it a significant risk of death. The surgery is also considered elective, because it is the patient who decides and it probably does not have to be done immediately.

Emergency surgery

While most decisions about surgery for UC are made over a time-scale that allows for careful thought and emotional adjustment, some operations have to be undertaken at very short notice. Such emergency surgery is necessary for several reasons, all of which are uncommon:

- toxic dilatation of the colon (megacolon);
- perforation of the colon;
- massive haemorrhaging of the colon;
- acute severe UC not responding to medical treatment.

Toxic dilatation of the colon is a condition in which the colon distends and is in danger of tearing. The symptoms are severe abdominal pain, nausea, vomiting, dehydration and high fever. It is not absolutely clear why toxic dilatation develops. It may be that there is a build-up of harmful bacteria that are producing toxins to such an extent that the colon's movements are paralysed, and so the faeces, bacteria and gas collect and cause the colon to swell. Alternatively, inflammation may be so severe that, unlike in most cases of UC, the ulcers go deeper into the colon wall, affecting the muscular layers.

If a tear appears in the intestine wall, some of the contents will escape into the abdominal cavity and cause peritonitis (inflammation of the lining of the abdomen), which can be life-threatening. This is why the development of a toxic dilatation warrants immediate surgical removal of the colon.

Similarly, if the colon is perforated (with a small hole appearing) emergency surgery is required. A perforation can occur if an abscess (infected ulcer) develops on the wall of the intestine or, very occasionally, during a colonoscopy, particularly if the colon has narrowed because of severe inflammation.

Haemorrhage is the medical term for bleeding. It is common for the colonic mucosa (inner lining) to bleed as a result of UC. If the inflammation becomes very severe, the bleeding may also become severe. On rare occasions the bleeding can be so severe that the patient is in danger of death, necessitating an emergency colectomy.

The fourth reason for emergency surgery is when UC has become so severe that the person has to be admitted to hospital for intensive treatment, which usually includes intravenous steroids. If the patient's condition does not improve after a few days, and particularly if it deteriorates, the decision may be made to operate. This last reason for emergency surgery is by far the most common. The other three are rare occurrences.

In all of the above examples of emergency surgery, the patient's written permission will be required. If, however, the patient is not in a fit state to make a reasoned decision then permission will be sought from the next of kin.

Elective surgery

With elective surgery your surgeon will recommend a particular type of operation, although more than one option may be available and you are likely to be asked for your preference. The different types of operation for UC all involve complete removal of the colon. This is because, if part of the colon remains, the inflammation may reappear in a part that is currently unaffected. Also, in cases of severe UC, there is continuing risk of developing colon cancer.

There are two main types of surgery. The difference between the two types focuses on what is done with the end of the small intestine once the colon has been removed. The small intestine is either:

- brought to the surface of the skin on the abdomen, forming an ileostomy; or
- fashioned into a small reservoir – an internal pouch – which is attached to the anus.

Many people would prefer an internal pouch because there is no obvious change to the appearance of the body, except for a scar. This is not always possible, however, and an ileostomy has to be formed instead. Many people are surprised at how quickly they get used to having an ileostomy, and some give the protruding intestine a name, as a way of coming to terms psychologically with the change in the appearance of their abdomen. Further information on pouches and ileostomies is given in the next chapter.

Specific surgical operations for ulcerative colitis

There are two main types of surgical operation for UC.

Proctocolectomy with ileostomy

This operation has been undertaken by surgeons for many years. Although the name of this operation sounds complicated, it can be easily understood by breaking it down into different parts. 'Ectomy' means the surgical removal of something. A colectomy is the removal of the colon. 'Procto' means anus or rectum, so a proctocolectomy is the surgical removal of the anal canal, the rectum and the colon. 'Ostomy' means the formation of a new opening. When the opening is for the ileum (the lower end of the small intestine) to pass through, the operation is known as an ileostomy.

A 'proctocolectomy with ileostomy' is therefore the removal of the colon, together with the rectum and the anal canal, and the formation of an opening in the abdomen through which the ileum protrudes (by a few centimetres).

The advantage of this operation is that there is no part of the intestine remaining in which UC inflammation can take place. Surgeons therefore describe it as a 'cure' for UC. As a straightforward operation it is less likely, compared with a pouch operation (described below), to cause complications either during or after the procedure. The main disadvantage is that the appearance of the body has been changed because a small pinky-red piece of intestine is permanently protruding from the abdomen. Also, it becomes necessary to learn how to manage the ileostomy with the use of stoma bags.

Colectomy with ileoanal pouch

This entails the removal of the colon and the fashioning of a reservoir (known as a pouch) from the end of the ileum, and attaching it to the anus. This is a more complicated operation, but in recent years it has become more commonly used for people with UC.

The main advantage of a 'colectomy with ileoanal pouch' is that a permanent ileostomy is not required. One disadvantage is that it is usually a two- or three-stage operation, involving a temporary ileostomy, with a gap of several months between each operation. Also, there tend to be more complications arising from the pouch compared with a permanent ileostomy.

In about 10 per cent of people with an inflamed colon, it is not possible to determine whether it is UC or Crohn's disease. This is described as 'indeterminate colitis'. An internal pouch is not recommended for people with Crohn's disease because inflammation may develop in the small intestine leading to the need for further surgery, which will disturb the pouch. Similarly, with indeterminate colitis an internal pouch operation will not be undertaken in case the illness proves to be Crohn's disease.

Other operations

There are two other operations for UC that are undertaken occasionally. If emergency surgery is needed, it usually is performed as a 'colectomy with ileostomy' in which the colon is removed, the rectum and anal canal remain, and a temporary ileostomy is formed. Once the patient has recovered fully, a decision can be made to remove the rectum and anal canal and make it a permanent ileostomy, or to keep the rectum and anal canal and form an ileoanal pouch.

Another operation, called a 'colectomy with ileorectal anastomosis', is performed rarely. This involves the removal of the colon, leaving the rectum and the anal canal. The ileum is then connected directly to the rectum. An anastomosis is the joining of two cut ends. This operation is only suitable for those with little or no inflammation of the rectum, which is rare in cases of UC.

Meeting the surgeon

If you decide to have surgery, you will meet a surgeon who will explain the operation to you. If there is anything that is not clear, do ask. This is not always easy – you may not remember the questions you wished to ask or be able to think up new ones in response to the doctor's explanation. Also, senior doctors can appear very busy and you may be reluctant to take up too much of their time. You, however, are the patient of the surgeon who has a duty of care towards you, so do take courage and engage in a conversation. It may be helpful to write down a list of questions beforehand.

Most people appear to be happier the more information they have. This is not true of everyone, however. Details about surgical operations can lead some people to worry more than if they simply put their trust in the skills of the surgeon. Each person is different and such differences need to be respected.

If you are a relative or close friend of someone who has UC, you may need to consider whether the person facing the operation really wants a lot of information. It may be that he or she is seeking reassurance from the surgeon, rather than wishing to be given all the details about the operation. To increase the likelihood that the meeting with the surgeon goes well, you, as a friend or relative, may need to think about what the person facing the surgery will be looking for.

If an ileostomy is to be formed, whether permanent or temporary, the patient will also meet a stoma care nurse or a colorectal nurse specialist. The nurse will provide advice and support for managing the ileostomy after the operation.

Going into hospital

Julia
Before I was admitted I had to have tests to check I was fit enough to go through with the surgery. It didn't feel that it was really going to happen, despite going home with a big black marker pen dot where my stoma was to be! It was only when I had to go on to the ward the day before admission to pick up some Picolax® (bowel cleanser) that it really hit me. I was frightened – very frightened. Not only of the surgery, but the stay in hospital and what the future would be like. I almost convinced myself that carrying on as I was wasn't that bad an option! Once actually in the hospital I gave up all these thoughts and just got swept along with it all, and before I knew it I was outside the operating theatre. Seeing the surgeon and all the other operating team was reassuring; I felt it was going to be all right. My last words before going under the anaesthetic were 'goodbye bowel'. It suddenly felt quite exciting!

Before the operation, the hospital will give you written information about what to bring into hospital (such as nightclothes and toiletries), and how to prepare yourself. You will be asked not to eat or drink (except for water) for a period before the operation. Also, you may have to drink a bowel cleanser (or bowel preparation), which is a strong laxative, in order to clear out all the remaining faeces.

On being accepted as an in-patient, before surgery, you will have your general health checked by a doctor. He or she will be looking for any signs of infection or illness (other than UC) that might mean that the surgery would have to be postponed. The information, including temperature, blood pressure and pulse, will also be used as base figures against which your post-operative recovery is measured.

If an ileostomy is to be performed, the stoma care nurse will make a mark on your abdomen where the surgeon will make the stoma. The nurse will discuss with you where the position should be.

You will also be asked to sign a consent form, which provides legal confirmation that you agree to the surgery being performed. The operation will not take place if the form is not signed. If, at the last moment, you decide that you do not want the operation to proceed, you should not sign the consent form. Obviously, however, it is very disruptive (and costly) for the hospital if you change your mind at the last moment. It is important, therefore, that you give careful thought to the surgery beforehand and are of a firm mind on the matter.

Assuming that you are proceeding with the surgery, an anaesthetist will explain how he or she will make you unconscious for the operation and how pain will be controlled afterwards.

Elise

I could not reduce my steroid doses very far without relapsing and, after trying all of the drug combinations, my specialist referred me to a surgeon. It was decided that I would have a colectomy with ileostomy. I cannot even begin to describe my feelings at this time; I was very frightened and could not believe that I would have to go through this at the age of 21.

My day of admission came round very quickly and as I prepared my bowels for the surgery, I became even more worried about what was going to take place the next day, but I kept reminding myself of how terrible my life had been before and that I did not want to be operated on as an emergency (which I had been told would almost certainly happen if I waited much longer).

I woke up the next day and got ready to go down to theatre. I said a very tearful goodbye to my parents and began what seemed like a never-ending walk to where my anaesthetist was standing, waiting for me. I climbed on the bed and he put my epidural in before sending me off to sleep, and the next thing that I remember was waking up in recovery attached to a drip and a catheter. The first week post-op was difficult as my bowels went on strike and my epidural hadn't been put in properly, but every week after that, things got significantly easier. At my follow-up appointment at the outpatients' clinic, my surgeon informed me that I now have nine years to decide whether I'd like to have the internal pouch or make my ileostomy permanent.

I soon saw what a positive difference my operation had had. I was no longer in pain or chained to the toilet! More importantly after living in what I can only describe as hell for four and a half years, I could finally start to live and have the sort of life that other people my age have! I can now see a future for myself, whereas before the surgery I couldn't, as I was always so ill.

Following the operation, you will probably regain consciousness in the recovery room, which is near to the operating theatre. Your condition will be closely monitored. Subsequently you will be moved to a room or ward in the hospital where you will recuperate.

To start with, you will have a number of tubes coming out of various parts of your body, either supplying fluids or drugs, or draining urine and bodily secretions. Pain relief will probably be provided by a tube directly into a vein. It may also be provided by an epidural, in which a fine needle is placed in the back. As you recover, you are more likely to have 'patient-controlled analgesia' whereby you can control the amount of painkiller delivered. There is a safety lock to prevent overdosing.

After a few days you will be allowed to drink water. Food will be gradually reintroduced some days later. Initially the food will be soft, liquid and easily digestible.

The various tubes will be removed, one by one, and painkillers may be taken by mouth. You will already be receiving an anticoagulant drug to reduce the risk of blood clots and you will be encouraged to get out of bed and take a walk, even though you may not feel ready to do so.

If you have an ileostomy, the stoma care nurse will visit you and show you how to look after the stoma (attaching the collection bag and emptying it when full). Generally an ileostomy bag is emptied four or five times a day and the bag is changed two or three times a week. This may seem a daunting challenge at first, but you will gradually get used to managing it.

It is not uncommon for people to feel depressed after an operation, perhaps because the body has gone through such a shocking experience. Usually this feeling passes, but if your depression persists, you could seek help from the hospital team responsible for your care. Relatives and friends can also be very supportive. And the patients' association *ia* (the Ileostomy and Internal Pouch Support Group) has trained visitors who can share their experience of having an ileostomy or an internal pouch (see Sources of help, p. 100).

Coming out of hospital

The length of stay in hospital depends on the type of operation and how ill you were when you first went in. For most patients who have had a colectomy, their stay in hospital is between 10 and 14 days.

The hospital will give you guidance on what you can do when you return home. You will be advised to avoid heavy work (such as lifting, ironing or vacuuming) until your wounds have healed and you have regained your strength. You may not be able to drive for a month or more and may not return to work for at least a couple of months. The time taken to recover will depend on the type of operation, your age, what type of work you do and your general state of health.

If you have had an operation for an internal pouch there will probably be a second operation (and sometimes a third), to complete the process. This will not take place until you have recovered from the first operation.

In the long run, the removal of your colon should make you feel a great deal better, because the UC will have finished. For a while, however, you may feel worse, because of the immediate effects of having surgery. You are likely to feel weak and tire easily. Furthermore, it will take time for you to get used to the ileostomy or the internal pouch. If you are having trouble with either do seek guidance from your stoma care nurse. He or she is there to help you.

In order to accelerate your recovery, you might want to undertake gentle exercise. Your doctor may be able to suggest a plan for this.

8

Living with an ileostomy or a pouch

If you are thinking about having a colectomy (surgical removal of the colon) it may be helpful to consider what life will be like with an ileostomy or an internal pouch.

If the ileum (lower small intestine) were to be connected directly to the anal canal, the semi-liquid contents would be hard to control and there would be a frequent need to go to the toilet. There would also be a worry about having an 'accident'. This is because having semi-liquid intestinal content is like being halfway between having properly formed stools and having liquid diarrhoea.

The difficulty in controlling one's bowels after removal of the colon is the main reason why either an ileostomy or an internal pouch is formed. The internal pouch is the equivalent of forming a very small replacement colon out of the end of the small intestine. An ileostomy involves the forming an alternative to the anus, so that the waste material no longer passes through the back passage.

Before describing what is involved with an ileostomy or an internal pouch, it is worth clarifying the meaning of the term 'pouch', which may be used in different ways. Some manufacturers of stoma care products describe their collection bags as 'pouches'. As a consequence, some people with an ileostomy also use the term in that context. Those who have an internal pouch, naturally refer to it as a 'pouch'; hence the confusion.

In this book the term 'pouch' is used to mean only an internal pouch.

Ileostomy

After a colectomy, a person is usually left with an ileostomy. The ileum is brought through a stoma (opening) in the abdomen. Instead of bodily waste passing through the anus, it comes out through the stoma and is collected in a bag, which is attached to the abdomen. An ileostomy is permanent unless an internal pouch is to be completed in a subsequent operation.

The protruding intestine of an ileostomy is moist and red. It looks as if it should be tender, but in fact it has no feeling because it contains no nerve endings. It can be touched without harm, although as with all openings to the body it is advisable to keep it clean and to wash your hands before touching it.

The ileostomy sticks out several centimetres. This is to avoid damage to the skin if the contents, which may contain irritating enzymes, leak out.

An ileostomy is usually placed on the lower right-hand side of the abdomen (below the navel), since that is near the end of the small intestine. Although this is approximately where the stoma will be made, there is scope for choosing the precise place within that area. The position of an ileostomy should be so that:

- you can see it;
- it is accessible in sitting, standing and lying positions;
- it does not get in the way of your usual clothing (for example, a trouser belt); and
- it avoids other parts of the body (for example, scars, the navel and abdominal fat creases).

By carefully considering such matters, the likelihood of having to reposition the stoma at a later date is decreased. The stoma care nurse will give advice on positioning.

When first created, an ileostomy will look bigger than it will subsequently. No waste will be produced for a few days, and then a semi-liquid content will be excreted. Unlike the anus, an ileostomy has no sphincter muscles. It is, therefore, not possible to control the time when the waste contents are pushed out from the body into the ileostomy bag.

The bag will initially be attached by a nurse, and emptied by him or her when it is full. Gradually, as you recover, you will be encouraged to learn how to manage an ileostomy bag. It fits around the ileostomy and sticks to the skin. When the bag is full it is emptied into the toilet while still attached. The bag is reusable for several days before it needs to be replaced.

There are many variations of ileostomy bag, and most of them have a filter that releases excess gas and eliminates odour. One of the main challenges is to make sure that the opening of the bag is the right size. It should fit over the stoma sufficiently closely that there are no leaks.

Other issues to consider are the consistency of the excreted material, and the amount of gas produced. The content is usually semi-liquid, but the degree of liquidity varies depending on the food that is eaten.

There is no special diet for people with ileostomies. This is because the small intestine, through which digested food is absorbed, is intact. It is, however, sensible to reduce:

- excessive gas, by avoiding beans and cabbage-like vegetables, onions and fizzy drinks and by not gulping down food; and
- obstruction near the opening of the stoma, by avoiding hard-to-digest items such as sweet corn, nuts, celery and coconut.

Each person is different. If there is a food that causes you difficulty, it will be easier to identify it if you keep a diary of what you eat.

Because ileostomy waste is runnier than normal stools, a higher volume of liquid is lost. Make sure that you drink enough liquid, especially in hot weather, to avoid dehydration.

Sometimes an ileostomy moves, either prolapsing (sticking out more) or retracting (moving back into the abdomen). In either case it may be necessary to have a further operation to get it back to the correct position.

Despite these difficulties, most people find they can lead a normal life with an ileostomy. There are few restrictions on the type of clothing you can wear, because the bag lies flat. The ileostomy should not stop you from engaging in vigorous exercise, although caution may be needed in contact sports.

Julia

With the surgery over, my new life started. First I had to learn how to cope with the stoma. Seeing it for the first time was a shock. I was more frightened by that than the scar the length of my stomach! As soon as I was able, I took myself off into the toilet to deal with the stoma myself. I felt I had to do this in order to get back some control. On the positive side, I noticed the benefits of the stoma within days of the surgery. I was now able to take my time waking up. No more stab of pain and running to the loo. It was wonderful.

Internal pouch

An internal pouch (properly known as an ileo-anal pouch) is a surgeon-made reservoir fashioned from the ileum and attached to the anal canal and rectum. The internal pouch acts as a small, alternative colon. The main advantage of an internal pouch is that there is no external sign of the pouch, and you can go to the toilet in the usual way.

Rachel
Now, with my pouch, I choose when to go to the loo rather than my UC telling me when. It has been wonderful deciding when I go to the loo and I can wait and wait!

Once the two or three stages of surgery have been completed, it takes some time for the pouch to settle down. Initially, you may find that you have to go to the toilet as frequently as you did with UC during a flare-up. For up to two years, the pouch gradually changes. It gets bigger and the cells lining the pouch wall look more like colonic cells than cells from a piece of small intestine.

Julia
After about three months, the pouch was tested for leaks by means of a barium X-ray and, as all was well, the reversal of the ileostomy was carried out. The stoma had become quite manageable. Time to relearn old skills! The first few days after having the reversal were quite nerve racking. I had to be careful not to dash to the loo every time I got the urge to go. I had to let the pouch start to learn its new function! It was hard at times, having to cope with leakages, wind and some discomfort. You really wonder if it is ever going to work properly. I was determined that it was not going to get the better of me and take control like the UC had.

Now, just over a year after the reversal I feel I am in control. The pouch does have times when it tries to gain the upper hand and lets me know it is there, but generally I would say that life is pretty brilliant. I feel well, pain-free and in control of my body. I feel good about myself again. I haven't felt this confident since before UC. The function of the pouch continues to improve and I hope it will do so for a while yet. I must admit I punish the pouch a bit with what I eat – anything and everything, but it is wonderful to be able to enjoy so many foods again without too much discomfort! The one downfall? I had thought I had escaped from having to dash into toilets at a moment's notice. But now it's not me – that's the joy of having a recently toilet-trained child!

As the pouch contents are more liquid than the stools in a colon, the sphincter muscles that control the opening and closing of the anus may not always be strong enough to stop some leakage, particularly at night when you are asleep. A protective pad may need to be worn until you have gained greater control of your sphincter muscles, which you can achieve through pelvic floor exercises. It still may be common, however, to empty the bowels between four and seven times a day, and night-time incontinence can affect one in five people with an internal pouch.

Failure rate for an internal pouch is low (between 5 and 10 per cent of patients, according to most authorities). A decision may be taken to have further surgery, this time to remove the pouch and form a permanent ileostomy.

Craig

For 13 years the pouch worked well. I ate and drank whatever I wished – including hot, spicy foods – without concession to my condition. I did, however, experience much tummy rumbling and some griping pain from 'wind' (particularly when running), which I could not always release safe in the knowledge that I would not 'leak'. In 1997, after suffering severe lower back pain for some time I was informed that my pouch had become septic and would have to be removed. For a while I was extremely upset, as the thought of wearing an external bag was daunting.

The ileostomy operation was performed and a whole new life opened up for me! After a few months of recuperation I went along to my running club, took a deep breath and explained to my friends what had taken place and asked if anyone would be offended if I changed and showered along with them as usual. To a man they were all very supportive and I resumed my sporting activities. However, I found I could now train hard (no griping pain etc., because the wind was automatically released into my bag) and I was transformed from 'one of the old, slow guys at the back of the field' into a runner who would figure in the club championship. I eventually became the second-division champion – beating many men much younger than myself.

I am able, now, to go into any sports complex and shower alongside complete strangers without embarrassment, although I try to be discreet and will walk with my towel in front of me, and shower facing the wall. My life continues quite normally – I merely use the toilet in a different manner to other people.

Another possible complication with an internal pouch is a form of inflammation known as pouchitis. The inflammation and symptoms are similar to UC. In most cases, it can be treated effectively with antibiotics, and there is also evidence that good-quality probiotics (which contain beneficial bacteria – see Chapter 10) may reduce the problem.

With any abdominal surgery, including surgery for an internal pouch or a permanent ileostomy, there is a risk of developing adhesions. Adhesions are scar tissue that develop in the area that has been operated on so that this area attaches itself to other parts of the intestine. Adhesions sometimes lead to kinks and twists that block or restrict the flow of content along the small intestine. The problem usually resolves of its own accord, but occasionally surgery is needed to cut away the adhesions.

Although there are difficulties with both ileostomies and internal pouches, it should be remembered that the person usually feels very much better after either operation, with no pain or fever and a lot more energy.

Sarah
Since the formation of my pouch, I lead an active life once more, which involves supply-teaching at the local primary school and enjoying socializing with friends and family. I imagined that I would always need to be near a toilet and could not comprehend it being possible to teach a class of children, travel on the motorway, or go to the cinema, pubs and night-clubs.

If there are any aspects of an ileostomy or internal pouch that are causing you worry or concern, you can discuss them with the stoma care nurse, who is likely to be very helpful and reassuring. Furthermore, there is additional help from *ia* (the Ileostomy and

Internal Pouch Support Group) or more detailed reading, such as the book *Living with a Stoma* by Dr Craig A. White (see Further reading, p. 104).

9

Special circumstances

Most of this book is relevant to everyone with UC. However, there are special circumstances for children and the elderly and in relation to reproduction. These areas are covered in this chapter.

Children

Approximately 15 per cent of people with UC are diagnosed before the age of 20, and most of these are in their teens. The symptoms, treatment and coping strategies for children and teenagers are very similar to those for adults, but there are some differences.

Younger children with UC report abdominal pain more often than adults, and a greater proportion of children seem to have extensive UC. Doses for drugs are adjusted downwards, according to the weight of the child. Steroids tend to be given more frequently to children to counter the more aggressive disease, but doctors also believe that it is very important to stop using steroids as soon as possible, because of the effects on growth and bones. Immunosuppressant drugs, such as azathioprine (Imuran®), are increasingly used in children as an alternative to steroids, because there are usually fewer side effects.

Anna

I am 13 years old and I got UC when I was 11 years old. I found out that I had it because of blood in my poo. It was getting worse, so my Mum took me to the doctors and they told me to starve myself for 24 hours because it could be a tummy bug. The starvation didn't work, so a few days later I went back to the doctor who told me to go to the hospital. They weren't sure what it was, so they did some tests on me, such as blood, temperature, pulse and an X-ray. Everything was all right, but as I had lost a lot of blood they kept me in overnight. The next day they said I could go home. A few weeks later I went back into hospital. They did a biopsy on me, and on the same day they found out that I had UC. I have been on and off steroids since and I am taking other drugs, as well as having lots of blood tests. Don't forget that there are people worse off than you. So UC doesn't seem so bad compared with some illnesses.

The main worry as far as children and teenagers are concerned is that growth and development is often slowed by the effect of the disease, the use of steroids and, sometimes, a reduced interest in food. The best way of overcoming this problem is to bring the disease under control and then to cease using steroids. This can be difficult to achieve in some children, and it may be necessary to supplement the diet by special nutrition.

A useful approach is to have elemental diet fed through a nasogastric tube. This involves the passing of a thin flexible tube through the nose and down into the stomach. The tube is connected to a bag of elemental diet, hung on a pole. The liquid nutrient is pumped automatically and slowly into the stomach, and as it flows into the small intestine it is absorbed into the body. This procedure usually takes place overnight while the child sleeps, and about 1000 calories are gained during that time. The tube is usually withdrawn in the morning, although some children prefer to keep it in place. Nasogastric tube feeding sounds unpleasant, but children tend to get used to it quickly and treat it as a routine activity. Before the tube is inserted, an anaesthetic spray may be used on the back of the throat to decrease discomfort and any tendency to retch.

Another way to increase growth is for the child to consume nutritional drinks as a supplement to the diet. These drinks, such as Ensure®, can be prescribed by a doctor, are available in a range of flavours and are reasonably palatable. They are packaged in small cartons, so the child does not look out of place drinking them at school or among friends.

In severe cases of UC, when the child has been taken into hospital, total parenteral nutrition may be used. Here, an elemental diet is added directly into a large vein, so that strength can be built up quickly.

Having a long-term illness can be a worrying and sometimes frightening experience for children. Hospitals will be unfamiliar places at first, so thought needs to be given as to how fears may be minimized.

One area of difficulty is undergoing numerous medical examinations and tests. Children with UC are monitored regularly to check development and disease activity. The tests can be frightening unless they are explained beforehand so that the child knows what to expect and can gradually learn to accept the procedures. The level of detail given will depend on the age and personality of the child, and parents will probably have a good idea how to approach the subject. The taking of blood for testing can be upsetting, and having an endoscope examination can be uncomfortable, embarrassing and sometimes frightening. There are special endoscopes for smaller patients, which may be more suitable for children. It is a good idea if a parent can be present during these procedures to comfort and reassure the child.

It is important that parents develop a good relationship with the doctors and nurses so that the hospital staff know about the child's particular circumstances. The staff may have special methods or ideas for making children comfortable.

Surgery is occasionally needed for children with UC. This needs careful thought. Removing the whole colon in a child or teenager is a major decision. Once the colon is gone it cannot be replaced, so the decision should not be rushed. On the other hand, if the child is suffering and medical treatments are not working, it may not be advisable to delay surgery.

If children have to have surgery, the aim usually is to form an internal pouch as the anal sphincter muscles tend to be stronger in children than in older people. Also, with a pouch there will be no external signs that the operation has taken place, other than a scar. In some cases an ileostomy may have to be formed, particularly in an emergency operation, but usually an internal pouch can be formed at a later date.

It is a good idea for parents to meet the child's schoolteachers to discuss the implications of their child's illness. A balance needs to be struck. On the one hand, reasonable allowances should be made for the UC, such as ready access to toilets and allowing a spare set of clothes to be kept at school. On the other hand, the child should, as much as possible, be obliged to follow the same rules as everyone else; and most children are keen to do this. If the child has to miss school because of illness, it is important to discuss with the teachers how he or she can avoid falling behind with schoolwork. Perhaps more homework can be provided, or a personal tutor.

As children move into their teens, they will want to be more independent. For example, they may want to be responsible for taking their own medications. They may also become rebellious and decide not to take the drugs consistently, especially if the UC is in remission. Managing such matters is yet one more challenge for parents as they help their child through the in-between stage of adolescence.

Parents may also need to think about how their sick child should be treated compared with their well brothers or sisters. It is not always easy to achieve a balance between properly caring for a child who is ill and treating all the children equally.

There are no hard and fast rules for dealing with these issues, because each family situation is different. It may be helpful, however, to get into the habit of having conversations over the dining table. Here family members can clear the air about misunderstandings, resentments and disagreements and sometimes be able to resolve them.

The over-60s

About one-fifth of all cases of UC are diagnosed in people over 60 years of age. Extensive UC is less common in this age group, while inflammation of the rectum and sigmoid colon only, or just the rectum, is more common. Nevertheless, despite the tendency for the disease to be less severe, the initial episode may be very severe.

Diagnosis is not easy, because the symptoms are similar to other bowel diseases that are common in older people. These include diverticular disease and ischaemic colitis. The latter is caused by a reduced supply of blood to the lining of the colon because the small arteries have hardened.

Diagnosis can also be delayed by a reluctance of some elderly people to report symptoms to a doctor, because they do not want to 'make a fuss'. This can be dangerous, because of the higher risks associated with the initial flare-up.

It is also more difficult to distinguish UC from Crohn's disease in the older age group. Difficulty in distinguishing between these two conditions occurs in about 20 per cent of older people, in whom only the colon is affected, while the figure is closer to 10 per cent in all ages. This difficulty is not a major problem, however, as treatment of the colon in patients over 60 is very similar for both those with Crohn's disease and UC.

Because older people tend to have more ailments, it is important that the doctor checks for potential cross-reaction between drugs for UC and those for other conditions. It is not always possible to predict such reactions, and so it is important to look out for unexpected side effects.

Corticosteroids can have debilitating side effects in older people. Emotional effects may be exaggerated, resulting in depression. There can also be a risk of developing diabetes, hypertension and osteoporosis. Steroids should therefore be used cautiously, particularly the systemic types. As with other ages, immunosuppressants may be used instead of steroids, particularly in difficult-to-treat UC.

Improving nutrition may be more complicated in older people. For example, it may be necessary to have a low-sugar diet because of diabetes, or a low-salt diet because of high blood pressure or heart disease. In cases of poor diet, particularly if there is insufficient nutrition, the advice of a dietitian should be sought.

John
With my improved health through switching to azathioprine, I decided to start running. In the same year as my sixtieth birthday, I ran a 10-kilometre race and a 10-mile race and participated in my first triathlon. The moral of the story is that no matter how ill you have been and for how long, you can always recover and tackle a new challenge.

Fertility and pregnancy

If a woman does not wish to become pregnant and is taking an oral contraceptive, there are two factors she needs to bear in mind. If she has severe diarrhoea, insufficient amounts of the contraceptive drug may be absorbed into the body, because the contents of the intestine are travelling too fast. Good data on this are not available, however, and the level of risk of the oral contraceptive failing is not known.

The other factor is that oral contraceptives slightly increase the risk of developing thromboses (bloodclots) in the veins, which may lead to an embolus (blockage of an artery). This risk is usually very low, but since people with UC already have an increased risk of thromboembolism arising from inflammation of the walls of veins, it may be advisable to use a low-strength oral contraceptive or use another method of contraception.

For those with UC who wish to have children, one of the first thoughts is whether the child will inherit the disease. Although UC does run in families, non-genetic factors are also involved in the cause. If one parent has UC the resultant child has about a one-in-50 chance of developing the disease. This risk increases substantially, to as much as one in three, if both parents have UC (or if one has UC and the other has Crohn's disease).

None of the medications normally used to treat UC affects female fertility, but there is one drug that affects male fertility. This is sulphasalazine (Salazopyrin®), which has been shown to alter the sperm count and the appearance and movement of sperm. Within two to three months of ceasing to take sulphasalazine, the sperm returns to normal. None of the other aminosalicylate drugs, such as mesalazine, have any noticeable effect on male fertility.

Most drugs used for UC do not have a negative effect on pregnancy. The more active the disease, however, the more the foetus (unborn baby) is at risk. Pregnant women with active UC are more likely to have a miscarriage, stillbirth, premature delivery or a low-birth-weight baby.

It is advisable, therefore, to try to get the UC into remission for at least three months before conceiving. If the disease is active at the time of conception, it is likely to remain active for the entire pregnancy, with the associated risk to the baby.

Pregnancy does not appear to increase or decrease UC symptoms. Also, the way that one pregnancy proceeds is not a predictor for how a subsequent pregnancy will proceed.

Christine
I have had two children who are now 25 and 22. I had no problems with pregnancy or labour. If anything, I remember feeling very well when pregnant. My first baby weighed 10lb 6oz and I always wondered whether that was due to the drugs I was taking (Salazopyrin® [sulphasalazine], Predsol® [prednisolone] enemas). But my second baby weighed 6lb 13oz, so there does not seem to be a pattern there.

There is no evidence that sigmoidoscopy induces premature labour. A colonoscopy does, however, carry more risk to the baby because of the need for a sedative before the procedure. A colonoscopy should therefore be avoided, as should the taking of X-ray pictures.

Evidence about the safety of UC medications during pregnancy is limited. This is another good reason to try to get the UC into remission at the beginning of pregnancy. Drugs that are believed to be safe include mesalazine, sulphasalazine, corticosteroids and the anti-diarrhoeal drug loperamide (Imodium®). Drugs that should not be taken while pregnant are methotrexate (an immunosuppressant drug), thalidomide (an experimental drug rarely used in UC) and diphenoxylate (an anti-diarrhoeal). Methotrexate should also not be taken by men while trying to induce conception because it affects sperm structure.

There are insufficient data on other drugs regularly used to treat UC to state with confidence whether or not they are safe for the foetus. In this group there are the immunosuppressants, azathioprine (Imuran®), 6-mercaptopurine (Puri-Nethol®) and ciclosporin (Sand-immun®). Most of the evidence on the use of azathioprine and 6-mercaptopurine in pregnancy has been from transplant patients. This has not shown any significant extra risks to the foetus. Many doctors will advise against trying to become pregnant when taking azathioprine or 6-mercaptopurine, but will recommend continuation of the drugs if they are already being used at the start of the pregnancy.

One study has suggested that complications in pregnancy are increased if the father has been taking 6-mercaptopurine during or up to three months before conception. The reliability of this study has been challenged, however. Currently there is no consensus on this matter.

Ciclosporin is effective with hard-to-treat UC. Evidence from transplant patients has been positive regarding pre-natal effects, although one study reported increased rates of low birth weight and premature birth.

Once a baby is born, the mother has to decide whether she will breastfeed or use a manufactured formula milk. It is safe to breastfeed if the mother is taking mesalazine or sulphasalazine. Corticosteroids are also considered safe in low doses, although with high doses there may be negative effects on the baby. The following are not safe to take while breastfeeding: methotrexate, thalidomide, ciclosporin, the antibiotics ciprofloxacin (Ciproxin®) and metronid-azole (Flagyl®), and the anti-diarrhoeals loperamide and diphenoxy-late. The evidence so far for the immunosuppressants azathioprine and 6-mercaptopurine is not sufficient to say whether they are safe or not with breastfeeding. If UC is active at the time of delivery, the mother may have difficulty producing enough milk for breastfeeding, because of her general physical and nutritional weakness.

If there is a serious complication of UC in the pregnant woman, such as severe bleeding, toxic dilatation of the colon or perforation of the intestine, emergency surgery should be undertaken to remove the colon. There is a risk of death for the foetus from the effects of the operation, particularly in the early stages of pregnancy. However, the mother's life is likely to be in danger if the surgery is not performed.

In men who are to have their rectum, as well as colon, surgically removed, surgeons take great care not to damage the nerves responsible for sexual function. Rarely, however, a man may become impotent. In women who have had a colectomy or who have an internal pouch there is some evidence of an increased risk of infertility.

Women with an internal pouch can have a successful delivery of their baby. The choice of vaginal or Caesarean delivery should be discussed with the doctor, since there are differing opinions as to which is better for someone with an internal pouch. Having UC does not of itself affect the decision whether to have a vaginal or a Caesarean delivery.

Annette

I was strongly advised to have a Caesarean section to deliver the baby as the pelvic floor and anal sphincter muscles are very important for a successful pouch, and normal delivery can put a great strain on these ... The Caesarean went well, except they decided to do a vertical incision rather than the usual horizontal one as they were concerned about the risk of adhesions from my previous surgery. This takes slightly longer to recover from, but wasn't too difficult to cope with and my days of wearing a bikini were over anyway due to my previous surgery! I had a beautiful baby girl on 20 December 2000 – the best Christmas present ever! I then went on to conceive again in 2002 and my second daughter was born by Caesarean in the same way on 12 February 2003.

The main problem I encountered was that immediately after I had my first daughter I was unable to locate my muscles to go to the loo for a few days and hence could not empty my pouch, which led to quite severe abdominal pain as my pouch got fuller and fuller ... I was able to go to the loo on the third day.

For my second pregnancy my obstetrician advised that they insert a catheter for a few days to drain the pouch until I could go myself. It didn't work brilliantly, but was enough to prevent the pain I had suffered previously.

For those with an ileostomy, there appear to be no extra problems with pregnancy. The ileostomy may block or swell, but this can be treated quickly and easily. Any change to the position of the protruding intestine usually resolves after the birth of the baby.

10

Probiotics and prebiotics

A subject that is generating a great deal of interest among people with UC is probiotics. These are products containing beneficial bacteria, which are aimed at achieving a better mixture of bacteria in the intestine. The idea of using 'natural' bacteria to counteract UC rather than 'artificial' drugs is attractive, especially because probiotics have very few side effects.

There are three reasons why probiotics are relevant to UC:

- the gut microflora (the hundreds of billions of bacteria resident in the colon) play an important role in the continued inflammation of UC;
- in the colon of people with UC, particularly in the mucosa, there is a different mixture of bacteria from that in people without intestinal disease; and
- there is growing evidence that the severity of UC can be reduced by consuming probiotic products.

The first point has been discussed earlier in the book, so let us concentrate on the other two points.

Attached to the mucosa (inner lining of the colon) there are many more bacteria in people with UC compared with healthy people. These bacteria are of the same types that constitute the normal microflora, except that there are proportionately fewer beneficial bacteria and more of the bacteria that are sometimes harmful (*Bacteroides* and *Escherichia coli*).

It is not clear whether this different mixture of bacteria in people with UC is a cause or a consequence of UC. It does, however, raise the question of whether, by increasing the numbers of beneficial bacteria in the colon, the severity of UC may be reduced. This has led to clinical trials using probiotics.

Clinical trials

A clinical trial studies the effectiveness of a given treatment in patients with a particular illness. Current evidence from clinical trials involves two types of probiotic, Mutaflor™ and VSL#3®.

Mutaflor™

Mutaflor™ contains a beneficial bacterium called '*Escherichia coli* Nissle 1917'. A German physician, Professor Alfred Nissle, discovered the bacterium during the First World War. He had been trying to discover why some soldiers in field hospitals were resistant to infectious diarrhoea, a common disease at the battlefront. By examining the stools of these 'resistant' soldiers, he was able to isolate bacteria that might be protecting against infection. In his laboratory, Nissle tested the isolated bacteria against typhus bacteria and selected the one that was most antagonistic to the disease-causing bacterium. After testing the beneficial bacterium on himself, Nissle produced Mutaflor™ to protect against gastroenteritis. It has been sold on the continent of Europe ever since, and is supplied in a capsule that is resistant to stomach acid.

In the 1990s, Mutaflor™ was used in two studies with UC patients. One study, involving 120 people with inactive UC, compared the effectiveness of Mutaflor™ with an aminosalicylate drug, mesalazine, maintaining remission. This 12-week randomized controlled study found there was no significant difference in the effectiveness of the probiotic and the aminosalicylate drug.

In the second study, 116 people with active UC received their standard treatment, plus Mutaflor™ or mesalazine, until remission was achieved. Then they continued with just the probiotic or the mesalazine for up to a year. There was no significant difference between the two treatments either in the proportion that achieved remission or in the proportion that maintained remission.

In a more recent study involving 222 patients with UC in remission, Mutaflor™ and mesalazine were again compared. After one year, there was no difference in the rates of relapse.

These three studies provide evidence for Mutaflor™ being an alternative to aminosalicylate drugs for the purpose of extending the period of remission from UC inflammation.

VSL#3®

Several controlled trials have shown benefit in people at risk of developing pouchitis (inflammation of the internal pouch). The probiotic used was VSL#3®, which contains eight species of bacteria that produce lactic acid, including two species that turn milk into yoghurt. The other six species are lactobacilli or bifidobacteria, which are types of bacteria that are broadly beneficial.

Lactic acid bacteria have been used for over a century as a food preservative (for example, in Italian hard sausages and sauerkraut). They have also been used for thousands of years in fermented milks, even though the cause of the fermentation was not known until the late nineteenth century.

The thinking behind VSL#3® is that a number of different bacterial species will have a synergistic response in which the combined effect is greater than the sum of the effects from each individual species. Also, compared with most other lactic acid probiotics, VSL#3® contains very large numbers of bacteria.

In one of the studies, 36 people with persistent pouchitis were brought into remission by two types of antibiotic, and then received VSL#3® or a placebo for one year. At the end of the year, 85 per cent of those receiving VSL#3® were still in remission compared with only 6 per cent of those receiving the placebo.

Current evidence suggests that antibiotics are usually effective at bringing pouchitis into remission and that VSL#3® helps to keep it there.

How do probiotics work?

It is not known for certain how probiotics work. It is, however, likely that they:

- increase acidity of the colon (through the production of lactic acid and other acids) that discourage the growth of harmful bacteria;
- attack harmful bacteria through anti-bacterial substances (bacteriocins);
- reduce gut permeability through the production of butyrate and other short-chain fatty acids, which improve the condition of the cells lining the colon;
- make it more difficult for harmful bacteria to multiply in the colon, by filling the vacant attachment sites on the lining of the colon (or by replacing the already-attached harmful bacteria); and
- decrease the production of pro-inflammatory chemicals by interacting with gut immune cells.

With any one probiotic bacterium, it may be that not all of these processes are involved in producing its beneficial effect.

Difficulties with probiotics

There are a number of difficulties with probiotics:

- they are currently not available on the NHS;
- the probiotics used in the clinical trials above are either not readily available in the UK or are expensive (or both);
- some products do not contain the same number and types of live bacteria as claimed on the packaging;
- although some products recommend a particular dosage, it is not clear whether that dose is sufficient to have an effect on UC inflammation;
- the fluctuating nature of UC means that it is not easy to be certain whether a probiotic product has worked.

Good-quality probiotics

What are the characteristics of a good-quality probiotic? Here is a suggested list of factors:

- a large number of probiotic bacteria;
- packaged and stored so there is a minimal reduction in numbers of live bacteria from the time of production;
- protected from the effects of stomach acid, either by special coatings or by the use of acid-resistant strains of bacteria;
- food mixed with the probiotic bacteria to help them live and grow as they travel through the intestine;
- containing species and strains that can attach themselves to the lining of the colon, to enable them to reproduce more easily and have a greater effect;
- containing species and strains for which there is some scientific evidence of health benefit;
- containing a mixture of probiotic species, rather than just one species, to increase the chances that at least one strain will be very effective.

To find out about the qualities of a particular probiotic, the first step is to read the packaging carefully, together with any associated leaflets. This will include information about the bacteria in the probiotic. The full name of a bacterium consists of three parts:

- the genus, such as *Lactobacillus* or *Bifidobacterium*;
- followed by the species, such as *acidophilus* or *longum*;
- followed by the strain (or variety).

The genus and species names are written in italics by scientists, although they are not usually italicized in probiotic product literature. Strains can be a name, a number or a combination. Many products do not give the strain details. Bacteria of the same genus have broadly the same characteristics, and those that are also of the same species will usually be even more similar.

The strain differences are usually quite minor, but occasionally a particular strain has a distinct characteristic that is especially useful in a probiotic. For example, the strain may be especially good at resisting the harmful effects of stomach acid, or very good at attaching to intestinal wall cells.

Some companies have a telephone helpline with qualified nutritionists or other scientifically trained staff to answer general enquiries from the public. Others have a website that gives further information about the probiotic. Some websites are little more than a way of promoting the product, but others carry a lot of useful information. Sometimes this information is kept on an area that is labelled as being for 'health professionals', but there is no reason why you should not read it. There may be information about the number of bacteria in the product, the characteristics of the strains, and any research that has been undertaken on those strains.

Consumer organizations and publications are good sources of information on probiotic products. Newspapers and magazines occasionally publish reports on the contents of probiotics, usually exposing those products that contain few beneficial bacteria. At the very least such reports can guide you on which products to avoid.

If, in consultation with your doctor, you decide to try probiotics, these are available from supermarkets, health-food stores, vitamin and mineral mail order companies, or direct from the probiotic companies themselves. Most of the probiotics available in supermarkets are milk-based, including live yoghurts and special drinks such as Yakult and Actimel®. Some fruit-juice probiotics, such as ProViva®, are also available from supermarkets. The probiotics from health-food stores and vitamin companies mostly consist of freeze-dried bacteria in capsules, powders or tablets.

Prebiotics

While probiotics enable the addition of desirable bacteria to the colon, another strategy involves the consumption of dietary fibre to enable the growth of beneficial bacteria already present in the intestine. This type of dietary fibre is known as a prebiotic.

Prebiotics are types of soluble fibre that can be found in the main body of some plants and act as a food store. Beneficial bacteria, especially bifidobacteria, find prebiotics easy to ferment and as a consequence they gain energy and nutrients and increase in numbers.

The best-known prebiotics are fructo-oligosaccharides and inulin. These are obtained from the root of the chicory plant. Fructo-oligosaccharides and inulin are also found naturally in bananas, leeks, asparagus, Jerusalem artichokes, onions and garlic.

Evidence of prebiotics improving UC is very limited. In a study on mice with colitis, a prebiotic was as effective as a lactobacillus probiotic in reducing the colitis.

In humans there have been three encouraging studies using different types of prebiotic. One study used lactulose (produced by combining sugars), another used 'germinated barley foodstuffs' and the third used fermented seeds of the Plantago plant. The last study was the most impressive: in 102 people with UC in remission, the Plantago seeds were as effective as an aminosalicylate drug in keeping the UC from relapsing over a 12-month period.

In another study, inulin was compared with a placebo in 24 people with pouchitis. All patients received both the inulin and the placebo, separately, and neither researchers nor the participants knew which was which. Inflammation was reduced during the time the prebiotic was consumed.

There are many other sources of soluble fibre that are being examined for prebiotic effect in boosting the numbers of beneficial bacteria in the intestine. Further research in this area can be expected.

There is one significant side effect with prebiotics: the production of gas, leading to bloating, abdominal pain and excess wind. This problem can be overcome by introducing a prebiotic gradually into the diet.

As with probiotics, there are no accepted recommended doses for people with UC. It should be noted that the amounts used in the four human studies mentioned above ranged from 8g to 30g a day.

If you decide that probiotics or prebiotics may help you and have identified one or more products that appear good quality, it is advisable to discuss your intentions with your doctor. People who are very ill, with a weakened immune system, may be at a higher risk of infection from the probiotic. Such infections are extremely rare, with only a handful of cases reported out of the millions of people who have consumed probiotics. Your doctor is highly trained and knowledgeable, and should have a good picture of the history of your illness. It is sensible to try to engage his or her interest and support in this non-standard approach. Many doctors will be very interested to hear what effect probiotics have on their UC patients. Furthermore, if your disease symptoms reduce as a consequence of the probiotics and prebiotics, you and your doctor will need to discuss any potential for reducing your other UC medications.

11
Future developments

It is natural to wonder what new treatments for UC might be available in the future, and how long it will take for a cure to be found. This chapter considers these areas of hope.

Genetics

Genes influence all biological processes. They are parts of chromosomes, which are strands of an extraordinary chemical called DNA. Chromosomes, 32 pairs of them, are found in every human cell. Each chromosome has thousands of genes, which instruct the body to develop and keep it maintained properly.

The gene responsible for a particular body activity will be almost identical in every human being. There may, however, be very small variations in genes between individuals that make the process they control work slightly differently. Some of the variations in genes may lead to disease.

The human genome is the total of all genes in a human being. The genome has recently been mapped and this has accelerated tremendously the study of the role of genes in human disease. It is only a matter of time before the genes involved in UC are identified. It is already known that UC is not caused by a single gene (unlike such diseases as haemophilia and cystic fibrosis, where if the gene is inherited from both parents, the child will definitely develop the disease).

Once scientists have identified the genes involved in UC, how might that knowledge be translated into improved treatment? The full consequences of mapping the human genome are hard to envisage. Here are some likely benefits in relation to UC:

- information about the types of genes associated with UC is likely to be extremely helpful in understanding what causes UC and how it develops;
- it will be easier to classify sub-types of UC and predict how the disease may develop within a particular person;

- drugs could be developed and selected that are targeted at the particular inflammatory processes involved in a sub-type of UC;
- relatives of people with UC could be assessed for their genetic susceptibility to develop UC and would be advised accordingly;
- clinical research should be able to involve a genetically similar group of participants, increasing the reliability of results and advancing medical knowledge more quickly.

Understanding the genetics of UC holds great promise, but this process cannot start until the specific genes have been identified and this may take several years yet.

Molecular biology

The study of genes is part of a science known as molecular biology, which is concerned with the molecules and chemical processes within living cells. Modern technologies have enabled molecular biology to be the most dynamic part of biology and offer the promise of greatly increasing our knowledge of UC. Our understanding of the cells and chemicals that constitute the immune system is growing. Tests on blood, tissue and stool samples can now provide more diverse information on disease activity, and improvements to such tests are likely to continue and accelerate.

Molecular biology is involved in almost all research on UC and has given fresh hope that the complicated processes involved in UC inflammation will be made clear. It also enables pharmaceutical companies to devise new drugs that will help to bring the disease under greater control.

Drugs

The main type of drug that has arisen from the investigations of molecular biology is known as a 'biologic'. The biologics are different from the current range of drugs for UC. They are either engineered molecules of specific chemicals within the inflammatory process or are aimed at targeting such inflammatory chemicals. For example, infliximab, a drug used for Crohn's disease, has been devised to neutralize a pro-inflammatory protein called TNF-alpha.

Currently, there are no biologics that can be prescribed for UC on the NHS, but there are several being tested on UC and showing early promise.

Other drug developments that can be anticipated include improvements to current drugs. Steroids and aminosalicylates are associated with a wide range of unpleasant side effects, mainly because they work systemically – that is, they pass from the intestine to the bloodstream and travel around the body. New types of these drugs are being developed that release the active component at or near the affected area, so reducing the potential for side effects.

Other aspects of UC research may provide an opportunity to develop drugs. The cells lining the colon are known to be more permeable to bacteria in people with UC than in healthy people. One product of bacterial fermentation, the short-chain fatty acid, butyrate, is absorbed and used by these cells. Butyrate enemas have demonstrated a positive effect on UC. Perhaps, as the cells become healthier by absorbing the butyrate, they also become less permeable and there are fewer gut bacteria provoking the immune cells to stimulate inflammation. Another way to strengthen the barrier function of the cells lining the colon may be the use of a protein, epidermal growth factor, which is found in saliva. Epidermal growth factor is known to help to heal wounds, and a recent study has suggested that it can also help produce remission in UC. It may be possible to produce drugs to supply butyrate, epidermal growth factor or some other agent that works on an important part of the intestine, such as the mucus that lines the colon.

Nicotine

One of the most extraordinary characteristics of UC is that, unlike most diseases, it improves with tobacco smoking. This is especially peculiar as the other main inflammatory bowel condition, Crohn's disease, is worsened by smoking.

Barbara
I had started smoking at 19 and only gave up when I married at the age of 25. Two years later on a trip to Paris, I noticed some blood in my stools and was diagnosed with proctitis.

The benefit of cigarette smoking in reducing the symptoms of UC is probably far outweighed by the harm smoking causes to many other aspects of health. It is therefore not recommended that people with UC take up cigarette smoking. It still may be possible, however, to take advantage of this peculiarity. It is the nicotine in tobacco that is the likely cause of benefit in UC, and it might be worth considering the merits of nicotine as an additional treatment for UC.

There have been several studies using transdermal nicotine (patches on the skin). Two good-quality studies in 1994 and 1997 involved a total of 136 patients with active UC. They received either transdermal nicotine or placebo patches (the latter containing no nicotine) for four to six weeks. All patients continued with their usual drug treatments at the same time. It has been calculated, by combining the study results, that one in four of the patients receiving nicotine had improvement in their symptoms that were almost certainly the result of the nicotine.

In a 1996 study, involving 61 patients with active UC, the benefits of nicotine were compared with those of a corticosteroid over a six-week period. While both groups benefited, the improvement using the steroid was greater. Smaller studies have suggested that the ability of nicotine to promote remission is enhanced when used in conjunction with aminosalicylate drugs.

In a study of nicotine as a maintenance treatment, 80 patients with UC in remission were given transdermal nicotine or placebo patches for six months. There was no significant difference between the two groups in the number who relapsed.

These results indicate that nicotine helps to bring active UC into remission, but has no benefit after that in keeping the disease from flaring up.

Are there any risks associated with nicotine patches? Most illnesses associated with smoking appear to be linked to the wide range of chemicals inhaled into the lungs. Nicotine is, however, a drug with a number of effects on the body. These effects are less addictive with skin patches, because by absorption through the skin the nicotine enters the bloodstream in a steady stream rather than in a sudden burst, as with smoking.

Side effects reported in studies in people with UC were nausea, light-headedness, headaches, sleep disturbance, skin rashes and tremor (slight shaking). These affected a substantial number of study participants. Using nicotine patches to help give up smoking involves starting with a high dose and gradually changing to a lower dose patch. With UC, it is probably better to move in the opposite direction, starting with a low dose and gradually increasing it, in case there are side effects. More than one patch should not be worn at any one time. In the future, controlled-release oral nicotine or rectal nicotine products may be developed that might have fewer side effects than transdermal patches.

It should be noted, however, that much is unknown about the long-term effects of nicotine, and the possibility of cancer-promoting effects cannot be ruled out. It is therefore important that you consult your doctor for more information on the possibility of nicotine treatment for UC.

Fish oil

Fish oil is well known for helping with flexibility and suppleness of joints. Less well known are its anti-inflammatory properties. Consumption of relatively large quantities of fish oil has been shown to reduce certain inflammatory cells and proteins and to reduce gut permeability.

These anti-inflammatory characteristics have led researchers to test whether fish oil is helpful in treating UC. Study results have been conflicting. Some positive studies have cited:

- a reduction in disease activity;
- an improvement in the microscopic signs of mucosal inflammation;
- a decrease in the amount of steroids used; and
- an increase in weight.

In other studies there was no discernable benefit.

The general picture is:

- no evidence of benefit in people whose UC is in remission; but
- some indication of benefit in people with active disease, particularly in allowing a reduction in the amount of steroids used.

Fish oil contains polyunsaturated fatty acids that are an essential part of human cells but that cannot be manufactured by the body. There are two types of polyunsaturated fatty acids: omega-3 and omega-6.

Fish oil products vary in the amount of omega-3 fatty acid they contain. The information on the labels may not give this information or it may be written in another form, such as EPA and DHA.

In research studies that reported positive responses in people with UC, the amount of omega-3 consumed each day was mainly in the range of 4–5.5g. This involved the consumption of between 12 and 18 fish oil capsules each day. In some participants there were side effects of fishy-smelling breath, belching and diarrhoea.

To overcome these side effects, one team of researchers tried an enteric-coated fish oil capsule, with the intention of protecting the omega-3 from stomach acid. Taking nine capsules a day (2.7g of omega-3), people in remission from Crohn's disease had significantly fewer relapses compared with the control group. No side effects were reported. It is to be hoped that similar studies using enteric-coated fish oil capsules will be undertaken on people with UC in the future.

Other advantages in taking fish oil may be a reduction in symptoms of joint inflammation and improvements in bone strength, since fish oil contains vitamin D, which aids the absorption of calcium.

As with all unorthodox treatments and dietary supplements, it is important to discuss the use of fish oils with your doctor.

Stress

Many people with UC believe that stress is a potential trigger for a flare-up. One study found that almost 40 per cent of their sample held this belief.

CW

I have had UC for 40 years and I have had only four major flare-ups in all that time. The first was at age 10 at the very start. The second was when I got married. The third was in 1992 and I cannot contribute the flare-up to any stress. I have no idea why it happened. The fourth was in 2000 just before my daughter got married.

There is evidence that psychological stress increases a person's susceptibility to illness and in people with UC long-term stress may have a greater influence over relapse than short-term stress. There is potential for further research in this area. In the meantime, people who feel that their UC is affected by stress should seek advice from their doctor on ways to reduce the stress.

Parasitic worms

Researchers from the University of Iowa, USA, tested the effectiveness of eggs of pig parasitic worms on people with active UC. Half the people received the worm eggs and half received a placebo (blank treatment), and then the treatment was crossed over. The combined results showed that 48 per cent of those receiving the worm eggs had reductions in the severity of their UC, compared with 15 per cent of those receiving the placebo. The parasitic worms were given in single doses of 2500 eggs every fortnight for 12 weeks. The eggs hatched into worms in the intestine, and on average it took six weeks for the maximum benefit to be experienced. There were no adverse effects from taking the worms, and they did not remain permanently in the intestine. It is not clear whether a product containing parasitic worm eggs will prove practical or attractive. However, this study does support the theory that the prevalence of UC in Western industrialized countries is due to the sanitized environments in which people live. In developing countries parasitic worms are found much more commonly in the human intestine.

Faecal enemas

A gastroenterology team in New South Wales, Australia, has reported six cases of people with hard-to-treat UC who have obtained complete remission through faecal enemas. Before starting the enema treatment, all of the patients took a course of antibiotics, followed by a bowel preparation to clean out the colon. They then received an enema solution of the faecal matter of a relative or close friend, whose faeces had been checked for any infectious microbes. Each person receiving the liquid enema had to hold it in for six to eight hours. The enema treatment was repeated for a further four consecutive days. There was no additional enema treatment after that.

All six people went into remission, and after several months they were able to cease all their medications. Subsequently, none of the six has relapsed, and at the time of the research report, the period of freedom from UC disease had been between one year and 13 years, depending on how recently the enema treatment had been given.

While this is not a controlled trial, and has not yet been replicated by other research centres, it does show that the prospect of finding a cure by manipulating bacteria in the colon is not beyond the bounds of possibility.

People with UC should remain optimistic that substantially improved treatments are on the horizon. There is good reason to be hopeful.

Glossary

Abdomen The part of the body containing the digestive and reproductive organs

Alimentary canal A tube that runs from the mouth to the anus, through which food passes as it is digested

Anal fissure A tear or cut near the anus

Ankylosing spondylitis An inflammatory disease of the spine that can also affect nearby joints, such as the hip, shoulder, neck and ribs

Anus Opening at the end of the alimentary canal through which solid waste matter leaves the body

Biopsy The removal of a small piece of living tissue for microscopic examination to discover the presence, cause or extent of disease

Bowels Another name for the intestine

Caecum The beginning of the colon, connected to the small intestine

Chyme Thick fluid that passes from the stomach to the small intestine, consisting of partly digested food and stomach secretions

Colectomy Surgical removal of the colon

Colitis Inflammation of the lining of the colon

Colon The part of the alimentary canal that follows on from the small intestine and has the function of removing water and salts from liquid faeces

Colonoscope A long flexible tube containing optical fibres that permit the examination of the whole of the colon

Constipation Difficulty in emptying the bowels, associated with hardened stools

Cortisol Another name for hydrocortisone

Crohn's disease A type of inflammatory bowel disease, similar to UC, but affecting any part of the alimentary canal, most often the small intestine

Diarrhoea The frequent passage of loose watery stools

Dietary fibre A general term for nondigestible carbohydrate in food, mostly from plant cell walls

Diverticular disease Formation of sac-like structures in the wall of the intestine that may trap particles of food or faeces and become inflamed

Duodenum The first part of the small intestine

Dysplasia The enlargement of an organ or tissue by the proliferation of abnormal cells

Elemental diet Nutritional liquid providing simple components that require no further digestion and are readily absorbed

Embolism Blockage of an artery by an embolus, which is usually by a blood clot or an air bubble

Endoscope An instrument for viewing the interior of a body cavity or organ

Enzyme A substance produced by a living organism that promotes a biochemical reaction

Epidural anaesthesia A painkiller introduced by injection near the spinal cord

Episcleritis Inflammation of the white of the eye and the skin of the eyelashes

Erythema nodosum A skin condition consisting of reddened tender nodules under the skin found on the extremities of the body, such as the shins

Faeces Waste matter remaining after food has been digested; it is discharged from the bowels

Flatus Gas from the intestine that is passed through the anus

Gastrocolic reflex A strong peristaltic movement of the colon, which occurs after a meal and that prompts the emptying of the bowels

Gastroenteritis Inflammation of the stomach and intestine, usually caused by infectious bacteria or viruses, leading to vomiting, fever, abdominal pain and diarrhoea

Gut Another word for the intestine

Gut microflora The thousands of billions of bacteria that reside in the intestine, chiefly the colon, and that act as a barrier to harmful microbes becoming established in the gut

Haemoglobin A protein containing iron, responsible for transporting oxygen in the bloodstream

Hydrocortisone A steroid hormone produced by the adrenal gland, and used as a drug to treat inflammation

Ileostomy The surgical formation of an opening of the ileum on to the abdomen, through which faecal matter is emptied

Ileum The third and last part of the small intestine, after the duodenum and jejunum

Immune system The tissues and organs that protect the body against harmful organisms and other foreign bodies

Inflammation An immune system response to infection or injury, involving the flooding of blood and white cells to the affected area, causing redness, heat, swelling and pain

Inflammatory bowel disease The general term covering UC and Crohn's disease and other conditions of long-term inflammation of the intestine

Internal pouch A reservoir formed from the ileum and attached to the rectum, following a colectomy

Intestine The lower part of the alimentary canal, from the end of the stomach to the anus

Irritable bowel syndrome A condition involving recurrent abdominal pain and diarrhoea or constipation, but without inflammation or other signs of damage to the intestine

Jejunum The part of the small intestine between the duodenum and the ileum

Lactose intolerance A sensitivity to lactose (milk sugar) caused by the inadequate production of the enzyme lactase, leading to bloating, flatus, nausea, diarrhoea and abdominal cramps

Large intestine Another name for the colon

Leucocyte A white blood cell

Microflora The microbes of a particular habitat, such as the intestine

Mucosa The inner lining of the intestine that secretes mucus as a form of protection

Mucus A slimy substance secreted by certain tissues

Nasogastric tube A thin plastic tube passed through the nose, down the oesophagus and into the stomach, in order to add or remove substances

Osteoporosis Loss of bone density, with an increased risk of fracture

Pancolitis UC affecting the whole colon

Patient-controlled analgesia A drug-delivery system that dispenses a preset dose of a painkiller when the patient presses a switch on an electric cord

Peristalsis Rhythmic muscle contractions that create a wave-like movement of the contents through the alimentary canal

Polyp A small growth, usually with a stalk, protruding from the mucosa

Prebiotics Food ingredients and supplements that encourage the growth of beneficial bacteria in the intestine

Primary sclerosing cholangitis A chronic inflammation of the bile ducts

Probiotics Foods or food supplements that contain beneficial bacteria, used with the intention of altering the mixtures of bacteria in the gut microflora and improving health as a consequence

Proctitis UC that affects just the rectum

Proctocolectomy The removal of the colon, rectum and anal canal

Proctosigmoiditis UC that affects just the rectum and sigmoid colon

Pus A thick yellowish or greenish liquid, usually consisting of dead white blood cells and bacteria, arising from the inflammatory process

Pyoderma gangrenosum A skin disease characterized by irregular boggy blue–red ulcers

Rectum The final section of the large intestine, between the sigmoid colon and the anus

Sacroiliitis Inflammation of bones in the lower back, causing stiffness and pain

Sigmoidoscope A tubular instrument, with a light at one end, used to examine the rectum and sigmoid colon

Stoma A surgically created opening of a hollow organ to the surface of the body, especially of the intestine on to the abdomen

Stools Solid faeces

Tenesmus False urges to evacuate the bowel

Total parenteral nutrition The delivery of a nutrient solution intravenously

Toxic dilatation of the colon A condition in which the peristalsis of the colon ceases, leading to the distension of the colon, risking perforation

Ulcer A crater-like open sore on the skin or on a mucus membrane

Ulcerative colitis (UC) A type of inflammatory bowel disease, similar to Crohn's disease, but affecting the colon only

Uveitis Inflammation of the iris, the coloured part of the eye

Sources of help

UK associations

The Bladder and Bowel Foundation
SATRA Innovation Park
Rockingham Road
Kettering
Northants NN16 9JH
Tel: 01536 533255 (general enquiries); 0845 345 0165 (nurse helpline for medical advice); 0870 770 3246 (counsellor helpline)
E-mail: info@bladderandbowelfoundation.org
Website: http://www.bladderandbowelfoundation.org

Core
3 St Andrews Place
London NW1 4LB
(enclose a stamped addressed envelope stating information required)
Tel: 020 7486 0341
Fax: 020 7224 2012
E-mail: info@corecharity.org.uk
Website: http://www.corecharity.org.uk

Crohn's in Childhood Research Association (CICRA)
Parkgate House
356 West Barnes Lane
Motspur Park
Surrey KT3 6QJ
Tel: 020 8949 6209
Fax: 020 8942 2044
E-mail: support@cicra.org
Website: http://www.cicra.org

IA – the Ileostomy and Internal Pouch Support Group
Peverill House
1–5 Mill Road
Ballyclare
Co Antrim BT39 9DR

Tel: 028 9334 4043; 0800 0184 724 (free)
Fax: 028 9332 4606
E-mail: info@iasupport.org
Website: http://www.the-ia.org.uk

National Association for Colitis and Crohn's Disease (NACC)
4 Beaumont House
Sutton Road
St Albans
Herts AL1 5HH
Tel: 01727 844296 or 0845 130 2233 (information line)
Fax: 01727 862550
E-mail: nacc@nacc.org.uk
Website: http://www.nacc.org.uk

RADAR
12 City Forum
250 City Road
London EC1V 8AF
(National key scheme for access to disabled toilets)
Tel: 020 7250 3222
Fax: 020 7250 0212
E-mail: radar@radar.org.uk
Website: http.//www.radar.org.uk

Overseas associations

Australia
Australian Crohn's and Colitis Association (ACCA)
Level 1, 462 Burwood Road
(PO Box 2160)
Hawthorn VIC 3122
Australia
Tel: +61 3 9815 1266
Fax: +61 3 9815 1299
E-mail: info@acca.net.au
Website: http://www.acca.net.au

Canada
Crohn's and Colitis Foundation of Canada
600–60 St Clair Avenue East
Toronto
Ontario M4T 1N5
Canada
Tel: +1 416 920 5035
Fax: +1 416 929 0364
E-mail: ccfc@ccfc.ca
Website: http://www.ccfc.ca

France
Association François Aupetit (AFA)
La Maison des MICI
78 quai de Jemmapes
75010 Paris
France
Tel: +33 1 43 07 00 49
Fax: +33 1 49 28 31 89
E-mail: info-accueil@afa.asso.fr
Website: http://www.afa.asso.fr

Germany
Deutsche Morbus Crohn/Colitis ulcerosa Vereinigung DCCV e.V.
Paracelsusstrasse 15
DE 51375 Leverkusen
Germany
Tel. +49 214 87608 0
Fax +49 214 87608 88
E-mail: info@dccv.de
Website: http://www.dccv.de

Ireland
Irish Society for Colitis and Crohn's Disease (ISCC)
Carmichael Centre
North Brunswick Street
Dublin 7
Ireland

Tel: +353 1 8721416
Fax: +353 1 8735737
E-mail: info@iscc.ie
Website: http://www.iscc.ie

New Zealand
Crohn's and Colitis Support Group (CCSG)
PO Box 28487
Remuera
Auckland
New Zealand
Tel: +64 9 636 7228
Toll-free (within NZ): 0508 227469
E-mail: ccsg@clear.net.nz
Website: http://www.ccsg.org.nz

United States of America
Crohn's and Colitis Foundation of America
386 Park Avenue South
17th Floor
New York
NY 10016
USA
Tel: +1 800 932 2423
E-mail: info@ccfa.org
Website: http://www.ccfa.org

Further reading

Jonathan Brostoff and Linda Gamlin, *The Complete Guide to Food Allergy and Intolerance*, Bloomsbury, London, 1998.

Dr Fred Saibil, *Crohn's Disease and Ulcerative Colitis*, Constable and Robinson, London, 2003.

Stephanie Zinser, *The Good Gut Guide*, Thorsons, London, 2003.

Stanley H. Stein and Richard P. Rood, *Inflammatory Bowel Disease*, Lippincott, Williams and Wilkins, Philadelphia, 1999.

Dr Joan Gomez, *Living with Crohn's Disease*, Sheldon Press, London, 2000.

Dr Craig A. White, *Living with a Stoma*, Sheldon Press, London, 1997.

Peter Cartwright, *Probiotics for Crohn's and Colitis*, Prentice Publishing, Ilford, Essex, 2003.

Cliff Kalibjian, *Straight from the Gut: Living with Crohn's Disease and Ulcerative Colitis*, O'Reilly and Associates, Sebastopol, California, 2003.

Dr J. O. Hunter, *The New Allergy Diet: The Step-by-Step Guide to Overcoming Food Intolerance*, Vermilion, London, 2000.

Index